Governance of HIV/AIDS

Nearly 30 years since HIV/AIDS was first identified, confusion over effective mechanisms of controlling and eradicating the illness remain prevalent. This book highlights the need for comprehensive approaches to governance, as responses to HIV/AIDS become increasingly focussed upon the health aspect of the epidemic, and financial commitments become subject to aid fatigue.

This book examines the roles and influence of multiple actors and initiatives that have come to constitute the global response to the epidemic. It considers how these actors and structures of governance enhance, or limit, participation and accountability, and the impact this is having upon effective HIV/AIDS responses across the world. The book addresses participation and accountability as key elements of governance in four thematic areas: the role of the state and democratic governance; non-state actors and mechanisms of political governance; public-private partnerships and economic governance; and multilateral institutions and global governance. Drawing on the insights of public health specialists, political scientists, economists, lawyers, those working with community groups, and within international organisations, it offers valuable perspectives on the governance of HIV/AIDS.

Aimed at both academics and practitioners throughout the world, this book contributes to the academic debate surrounding global governance, health and development economics, and the work of multiple international organisations and civil society organisations.

Sophie Harman is Lecturer in International Politics at City University, London. Previously she was Research Fellow at the CSGR, University of Warwick. She is the founding trustee of 'Trans Tanz', a Tanzanian-based organisation providing transportation to help rural communities affected by HIV/AIDS access healthcare facilities. **Franklyn Lisk** is currently Professorial Research Fellow at the Centre for the Study of Globalisation and Regionalisation (CSGR) at the University of Warwick, UK. He was previously a professor at the Africa Centre for HIV/AIDS Management, Stellenbosch University, South Africa; founding Director of the ILO Global Programme on HIV/AIDS and the World of Work in Geneva, and ILO Global co-ordinator for UNAIDS. He is the author of *Global Institutions and the HIV/AIDS Epidemic: Responding to an International Crisis* (also published by Routledge).

Routledge/Warwick Studies in Globalisation

Edited by Richard Higgott and published in association with the Centre for the Study of Globalisation and Regionalisation, University of Warwick.

What is globalisation and does it matter? How can we measure it? What are its policy implications? The Centre for the Study of Globalisation and Regionalisation at the University of Warwick is an international site for the study of key questions such as these in the theory and practice of globalisation and regionalisation. Its agenda is avowedly interdisciplinary. The work of the Centre will be showcased in this series.
This series comprises two strands:

Warwick Studies in Globalisation addresses the needs of students and teachers, and the titles will be published in hardback and paperback. Titles include:

Globalisation and the Asia-Pacific
Contested Territories
Edited by Kris Olds, Peter Dicken, Philip F. Kelly, Lily Kong and Henry Wai-chung Yeung

Regulating the Global Information Society
Edited by Christopher Marsden

Banking on Knowledge
The Genesis of the Global Development Network
Edited by Diane Stone

Historical Materialism and Globalisation
Edited by Hazel Smith and Mark Rupert

Civil Society and Global Finance
Edited by Jan Aart Scholte with Albrecht Schnabel

Towards a Global Polity
Edited by Morten Ougaard and Richard Higgott

New Regionalisms in the Global Political Economy
Theories and Cases
Edited by Shaun Breslin, Christopher W. Hughes, Nicola Phillips and Ben Rosamond

Development Issues in Global Governance
Public-Private Partnerships and Market Multilateralism
Benedicte Bull and Desmond McNeill

Globalizing Democracy
Political parties in emerging democracies
Edited by Peter Burnell

The Globalization of Political Violence
Globalization's Shadow
Edited by Richard Devetak and Christopher W. Hughes

Regionalisation and Global Governance
The Taming of Globalisation?
Edited by Andrew F. Cooper, Christopher W. Hughes and Philippe De Lombaerde

Routledge/Warwick Studies in Globalisation is a forum for innovative new research intended for a high-level specialist readership, and the titles will be available in hardback only. Titles include:

1. Non-State Actors and Authority in the Global System
Edited by Richard Higgott, Geoffrey Underhill and Andreas Bieler

2. Globalisation and Enlargement of the European Union
Austrian and Swedish Social Forces in the Struggle over Membership
Andreas Bieler

3. Rethinking Empowerment
Gender and Development in a Global/Local World
Edited by Jane L. Parpart, Shirin M. Rai and Kathleen Staudt

4. Globalising Intellectual Property Rights
The TRIPs Agreement
Duncan Matthews

5. Globalisation, Domestic Politics and Regionalism
The ASEAN Free Trade Area
Helen E. S. Nesadurai

6. Microregionalism and Governance in East Asia
Katsuhiro Sasuga

7. Global Knowledge Networks and International Development
Edited by Diane Stone and Simon Maxwell

8. Globalisation and Economic Security in East Asia
Governance and Institutions
Edited by Helen E. S Nesadurai

9. Regional Integration in East Asia and Europe
Convergence or Divergence?
Edited by Bertrand Fort and Douglas Webber

10. The Group of Seven
Finance Ministries, Central Banks and Global Financial Governance
Andrew Baker

11. Globalisation and Poverty
Channels and Policy Responses
Edited by Maurizio Bussolo and Jeffery I Round

12. Democratisation, Governance and Regionalism in East and Southeast Asia
A comparative study
Edited by Ian Marsh

13. Assessment and Measurement of Regional Integration
Edited by Philippe De Lombaerde

14. The World Bank and Governance
A decade of reform and reaction
Edited by Diane Stone and Christopher Wright

15. Nationalism and Global Solidarities
Alternative projections to neoliberal globalization
Edited by James Goodman and Paul James

16. The Evolution of Regionalism in Asia
Economic and Security Issues
Edited by Heribert Dieter

17. The World Bank and Social Transformation in International Politics
Liberalism, Governance and Sovereignty
David Williams

18. The Political Consequences of Anti-Americanism
Edited by Richard Higgott and Ivona Malbasic

19. The Role of Ideas in Political Analysis
A portrait of contemporary debates
Edited by Andreas Gofas and Colin Hay

20. Governance of HIV/AIDS
Making participation and accountability count
Edited by Sophie Harman and Franklyn Lisk

Governance of HIV/AIDS

Making participation and accountability count

Edited by
Sophie Harman and Franklyn Lisk

Routledge
Taylor & Francis Group
LONDON AND NEW YORK

First published 2009
by Routledge
2 Park Square, Milton Park, Abingdon, Oxon, OX14 4RN

Simultaneously published in the USA and Canada
by Routledge
711 Third Avenue, New York, NY 10017

Routledge is an imprint of the Taylor & Francis Group an informa business

Typeset in Times New Roman by Taylor & Francis Books
First issued in paperback 2013

British Library Cataloguing in Publication Data
A catalogue record for this book is available from the British Library

Library of Congress Cataloging in Publication Data
Governance of HIV/AIDS : making participation and accountability count / edited by Sophie Harman and Franklyn Lisk.
p. cm. – (Routledge/Warwick studies in globalisation; 20)
Includes bibliographical references and index.
1. HIV infections–Government policy. 2. AIDS (Disease)–Government policy. I. Harman, Sophie. II. Lisk, Franklyn.
RA643.8.G68 2009
362.196'9792–dc22
2008054936

ISBN13: 978-0-415-48564-7 (hbk)
ISBN13: 978-0-415-84802-2 (pbk)

Contents

Acknowledgements

The editors would like to thank the Centre for the Study of Globalisation and Regionalisation (CSGR), University of Warwick and the United Nations Development Programme (UNDP) for supporting this joint collaboration. We would specifically like to thank Joseph Annan, Violet Baffour, and Blerta Cela from UNDP for their input and support; and Richard Higgott and Diane Stone from the University of Warwick for introducing the two of us to each other, suggesting a possible collaboration, and supporting the various stages of preparing the book. Thank you to those who attended the two-day conference of the same name in November 2007, and the two book reviewers, your comments and feedback were extremely helpful.

Abbreviations

ABC	Abstain, Be faithful, use a Condom
ACT Africa	AIDS Campaign Team Africa
ADB	Asian Development Bank
AIDS	Acquired Immune Deficiency Syndrome
ANC	African National Congress
ART	Anti-retroviral Therapy
CAF	Community Action Fund
CBO	Community Based Organisation
CCM	Country Co-ordinating Mechanism
CDC	Center for Disease Control
CDF	Comprehensive Development Framework
CSO	Civil Society Organisation
CSR	Corporate Social Responsibility
CSW	Commercial Sex Worker
DAC	District AIDS Council
DFID	Department for International Development
FBO	Faith based organisation
GBC	Global Business Council on HIV/AIDS
Global Fund	Global Fund to fight HIV/AIDS, Tuberculosis and Malaria
GPA	Global Program on HIV/AIDS
HIV	Human Immuno-deficiency Virus
IAVI	International AIDS Vaccine Initiative
IDA	International Development Agency
IDU	Intravenous Drug User
ILO	International Labour Organisation
IMF	International Monetary Fund
INGO	International Non-Governmental Organisation
LFA	Local Fund Agent
MAP	Multi-Country AIDS Programme
MDG	Millennium Development Goal
NAC	National AIDS Council
NATF	National AIDS Trust Fund
NGO	Non-governmental Organisation

NUM	National Union of Mineworkers
OVC	Orphans and Vulnerable Children
PDP	Product Development Partnership
PEPFAR	President's Emergency Plan for HIV/AIDS Relief
PLWHA	People Living With HIV/AIDS
PMTCT	Prevention of Mother to Child Transmission
PR	Principal Recipients
PRSP	Poverty Reduction Strategy Paper
SABCOHA	South African Business Coalition on HIV/AIDS
SADC	Southern African Development Community
STI	Sexually Transmitted Infection
TACAIDS	Tanzania Commission for HIV/AIDS
TANs	Transnational Advocacy Networks
TASO	The AIDS Support Organisation
TRIPs	Trade-related Intellectual Property Rights
UAC	Uganda AIDS Commission
UN	United Nations
UNAIDS	Joint United Nations Programme on HIV/AIDS
UNDP	United Nations Development Programme
UNFPA	United Nations Population Fund
UNICEF	United Nations Children's Fund
UNIFEM	United Nations Fund for Women
UNGASS	United Nations General Assemble Special Session on HIV/AIDS
USAID	United States Agency for International Development
VCT	Voluntary Counselling and Testing
WFP	World Food Programme
WHO	World Health Organisation
WTO	World Trade Organisation

Contributors

Kondwani Chirambo is the Manager of the Governance of AIDS Programme of Idasa. He initiated this study on HIV/AIDS and Electoral Democracy in 2003. Kondwani holds an MA in Mass Communications, awarded by the Faculty of Social Sciences, University of Leicester. He is also currently studying for his PhD in the field of Communication Science with the University of South Africa.

Antoinette Handley is Assistant Professor in the Department of Political Science at the University of Toronto. Her research interests include policymaking and economic reform in developing countries, business-government relations, and HIV/AIDS and the political economies of Africa. Her book, Business and the State in Africa: Economic Policymaking in the Neo-Liberal Era, was published by Cambridge University Press in early 2008.

Sophie Harman is a Lecturer in International Politics at City University, London. She has conducted extensive research into World Bank-Civil Society engagement within the Multi-Country AIDS Programme in East Africa. She is the founding trustee of 'Trans Tanz', a Tanzanian-based organisation providing transportation to help rural communities affected by HIV/AIDS access healthcare facilities. Her primary interests are institutions of global governance, civil society, women's rights and gender, and HIV/AIDS governance.

Felicity Hatendi-Gutu is the outgoing UNDP Zimbabwe Global Fund Manager. She has an MSc in Strategic Management, BA in Adult Education, and holds several educational and professional qualifications in the health and development field. She is a local and Southern African consultant, trainer, programmer, researcher in the area of HIV/AIDS, health, and development.

Shannon Hayes has worked as the coordinator of the Huairou Commission AIDS Campaign and for GROOTS International in Africa since 2004. Shannon, working closely with GROOTS Kenya, has played a lead supportive role in the organization of the Home-Based Care Alliance in

Africa. She holds a BA in History from the University of California at Santa Barbara and a MA in International Affairs from The New School.

Franklyn Lisk is currently Professorial Research Fellow at the Centre for the Study of Globalisation and Regionalisation (CSGR), University of Warwick and was a Professor at the Africa Centre for HIV/AIDS Management, at Stellenbosch University, South Africa, from 2005 to 2007. Prior to that he was founding Director of the ILO Global Programme on HIV/AIDS and the World of Work in Geneva, and ILO Global co-ordinator for UNAIDS. He has published widely on the subject of the economic and social impact and governance of HIV/AIDS, and on globalisation and international development issues.

Helen Potts, PhD, is a Senior Research Officer in the Right to Health Unit, Human Rights Centre. Helen is both a lawyer and a public health practitioner. She has extensive field experience having worked in Australia (including Indigenous Australia), Thailand, Saudi Arabia, Papua New Guinea, Democratic People's Republic of Korea and Cambodia. Past research activity has been concerned with access to health care by marginalised groups. Current research interests include the nature of accountability in the context of the right to health, and the right of participation by individuals and groups in public health strategy development.

Dylan Sutherland is a Lecturer in the School of Contemporary Chinese Studies at Nottingham University. He has published in the areas of Chinese economy and development. He is now working on an interdisciplinary project exploring the economic and social determinants of HIV/AIDS in China.

Introduction

Governance of the HIV/AIDS response: Making participation and accountability count

Sophie Harman

The global crisis of the HIV/AIDS epidemic has been met with an unprecedented level of financial, political and personal commitment to address its spread, help those living with the disease, and address its roots in socio-economic poverty. This commitment comes with new forms of coordination and cooperation in approaching the dual problem of articulating what works, and how we approach the sensitivities of other people's sex lives in the context of shifts within the global political economy. The complexities surrounding the spread and impact of HIV/AIDS require a multifaceted approach to address this problem. Central to this approach is a structured form of governance regime that constitutes the global response to HIV/AIDS, and how to make this regime made up of multiple actors with different interests and approaches, accountable to people living with and affected by HIV/AIDS.

Commonly associated with effective means of service delivery and the leadership of governments, governance has been increasingly recognised as a central component in effectively realising an end to the impact and spread of HIV/AIDS. With the plethora of actors, regulations, and norms associated with means of responding to the epidemic, notions of governance, who is governing whom and for what purpose, have become blurred. Governments are still of paramount importance to tackling the epidemic in any particular country, and are thus central to any conception of governance in this regard. Yet, the emergence of civil society organisations (CSOs) – from small community groups to international advocacy organisations, private-public partnerships, informal networks, multilateral and bilateral donors, United Nations agencies and regional bodies challenges preconceived notions of governance as influence upon decision-making, agenda-setting and service delivery. Confusion as to who is doing what, who is influencing whom, and who is governing what amid structures of economic and social inequalities exists, at every level of the HIV/AIDS response, undermining any form of cohesion and cooperation in the face of this global crisis. These challenges lead to the crux of the problem within HIV/AIDS governance: participation and accountability.

The multiple actors involved within the response to HIV/AIDS suggest that widespread participation is not a significant issue. What is unclear, however, is what is meant by participation, who is participating and why they participate, and the outcome of this. Questions remain as to what claims to legitimacy these actors have, how legitimacy is fashioned within HIV/AIDS governance and the impact this is having on the disaggregated forms of alternative participation. Conceptions of legitimacy are bounded within mechanisms of accountability, and whether one infers the other. Accountability and structures of accountability have come to mean different things for different actors within the response. Accountability has become a tool of governance, in regards to who is able to hold whom to account, which actors remain unaccountable and why, and the gaps that exist in measuring accountability. Problems with accountability and participation have been central to the agenda of international organisations, governments, and donors within the HIV/AIDS response, but in practice these concepts are narrowly understood and thus unequally applied. These bodies demand structures of accountability and participation from those working in the field of HIV/AIDS and those infected with and/or affected by the disease; but they fail to reciprocate such levels of accountability and participation. As such, perceptions of what governance means in regards to HIV/AIDS remains problematic both in theory and, crucially, in practice.

This book unravels some of these issues, and confronts what we mean when we talk about participation, accountability and governance in regards to every aspect of the HIV/AIDS response. It does so by drawing on the work of public health specialists, political scientists, economists, lawyers, those working with community groups and within international organisations, to offer different and revealing perspectives as to what governance means in regards to HIV/AIDS and 'the response'. The eight central chapters of the book provide a snapshot of the multiplicity of actors involved within the response, problems of accountability and partnership, and empirical evidence as to how these problems unravel in practice. As such, the book addresses four pertinent areas of HIV/AIDS governance:

(i) role of the state and democratic governance;
(ii) non-state actors, popular participation and mechanisms of accountable governance;
(iii) partnerships: public-private, formal and informal Networks; and
(iv) global governance and multisectoralism.

Pertinent issues within the governance of HIV/AIDS, such as how to address the feminisation of the epidemic, is addressed within each of the chapters. As HIV/AIDS is a disease that disproportionately affects women, the book does not have a specific 'add-on' chapter confronting the issue of gender, but considers this issue as part of the epidemic as a whole. The purpose of this book is not only to demystify some of the issues surrounding HIV/AIDS governance, but to interrogate these structures, and the outcomes they are having on the people, communities and states affected and devastated by this epidemic.

The book is by no means a comprehensive account of governance, but provides a detailed exploration of some of the key issues, factors and means of understanding this concept in regards to HIV/AIDS.

Background to the project

Governance and HIV/AIDS: Making Participation and Accountability Count is the culmination of an ongoing partnership between the Centre for the Study of Globalisation and Regionalisation (CSGR), University of Warwick, and the HIV/AIDS Group, United Nations Development Programme (UNDP). The papers collected here are taken from the conference of the same name, held at the University of Warwick 5–6 November 2007. The purpose of the conference was to provide a focus upon HIV/AIDS that acknowledged its interconnectedness with development planning, outcomes and the capacity of individual countries to articulate and address their own interventions in response to the epidemic. The concept of the conference originated from the issues and concerns raised during the first phase of the CSGR/UNDP collaboration: (i) the elaboration of conceptual and methodological issues that underline the two-way relationship between effective governance and effective HIV/AIDS response at global, regional and national levels; and (ii) the preparation of three 'framework' papers on governance and HIV/AIDS response. The issues raised within these three papers highlighted the need for a more comprehensive approach to HIV/AIDS governance and dialogue and debate between a variety of academics and practitioners so as to identify the various conceptions, gaps and outcomes of HIV/AIDS governance. Held over two days, the conference sought to highlight innovative research within this field and draw from the collective experiences and opinions of different actors, with the overall aim of identifying the main barriers to effective HIV/AIDS response posed by governance structures past, new and emerging, and means of challenging these barriers. The book not only presents the outcome of the conference, but also establishes a basis upon which to start a conversation and build future debate and research surrounding the governance agenda and how we can begin to characterise the global response to HIV/AIDS in terms of governance and regime.

Thematic areas

The book is organised around the main thematic areas of the conference. The first area considers the role of the state and democratic governance. State structures, and the articulation and deployment of national development strategies that acknowledge and address HIV/AIDS directly at the highest level of government, are widely accepted as key to an effective response to the epidemic. In addition to the demands of managing the interests of donors, international and regional actors, and CSOs, the response to HIV/AIDS has seen a shifting of state practice in some countries to open democratic and participatory procedure. The wider impact of this upon democratic governance, and the promotion thereof, raises a contention between state sovereignty and influence, and the ability of people and organisations to hold the governments that represent them to account. Democratic practice is perceived as intertwined with effective deployment of funds, service delivery, tools to equip community-led responses to the epidemic, project design, feedback and monitoring and evaluation. The impact that this has upon states' ability to govern and lead the response, however, is of paramount concern. It raises questions as to whether the HIV/AIDS response is used as a vehicle with which to promote democratic practice, the legitimacy of this, its outcome, and how it leads to specific forms of governance; and the relationship between socio-economic inequalities within particular states and how we can understand this within specific contexts. As such, the purpose of this section is to explore questions of:

- Is there still a role for the government within HIV/AIDS?
- How have HIV/AIDS responses been used as a democratising force?
- What impact has HIV/AIDS had upon systems of governing within particular states?
- How have HIV/AIDS responses affected sovereign borders and the ability of governments to rule and direct their health systems?

The role of non-state actors, popular participation and mechanisms of accountable governance presents the second thematic area in which the book is organised. Emphasis upon multisectoralism within the HIV/AIDS response has contributed to a mushrooming of non-state actors at every level of decision-making and practice within the response. Non-state actors are now enjoying greater influence and representation in decision-making as a result of key initiatives such as the Global Fund to Fight AIDS, Tuberculosis and Malaria, the World Bank's Multi-Country AIDS Program, and the United Nation's commitment to a multisectoral response led by UNDP. Such inclusion reveals much about the presence of CSOs and the shifting dynamics of popular participation and renewed accountability mechanisms. The extent to which these organisations are involved in decision-making remains contentious, with coordination and collaboration remaining limited to certain actors, and the lack of capacity or mechanisms within state, regional and global structures of decision-making to fully harness and recognise the capacity and role of such actors. Crucial to non-state participation and mechanisms of accountability is the introduction of guidelines, legal frameworks and international agreements that commit actors to specific rights, justice and accountability within the HIV/AIDS response. There is a great need to recognise and articulate effective means to use or create wider mechanisms for inclusion, understanding, and coordination between the multiple actors involved within the response for it to work effectively. Pertinent to which are questions of:

- What role do non-state actors have within the HIV/AIDS response?
- Do non-state actors have the capacity to influence decision-making?
- Do non-state actors complicate or enhance delivery?
- What are the main mechanisms of non-state participation and accountability?

The emergence of public-private partnerships, formal and informal networks presents the third thematic area of concern. The increased existence of public–private partnerships, product-development partnerships, foundations and networks requires a renewed focus upon the role of the private sector within the HIV/AIDS response. Crucial to this is how states and CSOs can build relationships with private actors and utilise them effectively within national planning, delivery and sustaining long-term commitment to addressing the socio-economic consequences of the epidemic. The existence of these actors requires a balance between new forms of regulation and accountability and encouraging investment and provision, based upon positive discrimination and acceptance of people infected with and affected by HIV/AIDS. Inclusion of private actors and public-private partnerships refocuses the nature of governance and clear-cut divisions between the private and public sector. Forms of engagement such as informal and formal networks and collaborations have been a central mechanism in which non-state actors have influenced decision-making and policy within HIV/AIDS governance. Their capacity to reach a wide range of people and interests places them at the centre of the response, developing innovative and inclusionary practices for their employees that are often ahead of government practice. Often favoured as a means of inclusion within governmental structures of decision-making, networks are a key site for accountability mechanisms and governance, yet understandings of which are under-developed within the context of HIV/AIDS. Thus, the following questions remain important to any understanding of HIV/AIDS governance:

- How do formal and informal networks and the role of the private sector contribute to our understanding of HIV/AIDS governance?
- Do these networks promote or detract from effective HIV/AIDS governance?
- Do public-private partnerships run contrary to the objectives of governments/CSOs?
- What does the role of the private sector reveal about that of governments?

The final thematic area explored within the book is global governance and multisectoralism. The multiplicity of international organisations, multilateral donors, bilateral donors, and regional groups involved within the HIV/AIDS response has led to confusion about their competing mandates and coordination. Mechanisms such as UNAIDS' commitment to 'The Three Ones' – one strategic plan, one coordinating body and one monitoring and evaluation system – have been widely adopted, but limits to their effective use remain prevalent. Moreover, the presence and influence of such institutions raise questions over the nature and impact of their interventions in terms of how the response is governed, who is doing the governing, and how this contributes to wider understanding of global and regional governance. Focus upon the interrelationships between different global and regional institutions and states, their role within the response, and how they effect conceptions of governance in this instance therefore becomes of central relevance. At the forefront of this are questions of:

- Which global and regional institutions affect the governance of HIV/AIDS?
- What impact are they having upon the response?
- How are they working with non-state actors, governments and states?
- What ramifications do their involvement in HIV/AIDS have upon our understanding of global governance and international organisations?

As these questions and thematic summaries suggest, most of these issue areas are overlapping and interrelated. It is therefore important to consider these issues in light of several key questions that this book seeks to interrogate and use as its central basis for research:

- What is meant by governance in regards to HIV/AIDS?
- Who is governing whom to what end?
- What is effectiveness and how do we measure it?
- Should we make participation and accountability count?

Chapter breakdown

The book begins by concentrating on the role of the state and democratic governance within the HIV/AIDS response in regards to two distinct case studies: an intricate examination of six countries in Sub-Saharan Africa, and one of China. Kondwani Chirambo's chapter 'AIDS, politics and governance: The impact on HIV/AIDS on electoral processes' in Namibia, Malawi, Senegal, South Africa, Tanzania and Zambia' uses a comparative study to assesses the impact HIV/AIDS is having upon the electoral systems within these countries. The chapter carefully outlines the practical and long-term economic, social and political affect the epidemic has upon different forms of political systems, and in so doing offers recommendations and suggestions as to the betterment of existing systems and those that are more robust against the affects of the epidemic. Dylan Sutherland's chapter, 'Economic and social inequalities and HIV/AIDS in China: Implications for policy and governance' challenges the inter-relationship between poverty and HIV/AIDS within the context of China, to see how social inequalities are leading to the epidemic's growth. Based upon extensive field research, Sutherland explores different social explanatory variables, such as gender, to identify evidence as to the inter-linkage between the epidemic and inequality, and specific patterns in this relationship. Sutherland outlines specific regional indicators of this relationship, and then tests these indicators within thirty Chinese provinces. In so doing, Sutherland's chapter draws out how inequality, the state and the epidemic have become intertwined within China and how this relates to governance.

The second section of the book considers the role of non-state actors, popular participation, and mechanisms of accountable governance, looks at both the role of non-state actors and their relationship with governance by focusing on the work of the community-based Home-Based Care Alliance in Kenya, and the right to health as a mechanism of accountability within HIV/AIDS governance. Helen Potts' chapter, 'Accountability and the right of everyone to the enjoyment of the highest attainable standard of physical and mental health' engages with understandings of a right to health and how this can be developed by policy practitioners and those engaged in delivery. Fundamental to Potts' analysis is the pre-requisite of accountability within the realisation of the right to health, and its central role as a mechanism to accountable HIV/AIDS governance. Shannon Hayes' chapter 'The Home-Based Care Alliance in Kenya: Improving governance and transforming communities in the context of HIV/AIDS' offers an insight into the activity of those involved in service delivery, and the vital role of home-based carers not only in the delivery of services and support of people living with HIV/AIDS, but their role in improving forms of local and national accountable governance. Coming from a practitioner's perspective, Hayes is able to pinpoint the specific circumstances and capacity of the home based carers to hold local government authorities in Western Kenya to account and how they are able to move from service delivery roles to influence decision-making.

In the third section of the book, Antoinette Handley and Franklyn Lisk address the role of the private sector within the governance of the HIV/AIDS response. Antoinette Handley contributes to understandings of governance by focusing directly upon the role of business within the HIV/AIDS response in South Africa in the chapter 'Business and the governance of HIV/AIDS in South Africa'. Handley critically assesses the role businesses have had in responding to the epidemic, and in turn examines the impact the epidemic has had upon these businesses themselves. In this analysis, Handley situates the role businesses have had in the provision of care and treatment of employees in conjunction with the Government of South Africa's apparent inaction in response to the country's HIV/AIDS crisis. Handley explores some of the emerging effects that business provision of services may have upon stigma, status and job security, as well as the relative limitations such an interpretation of provision and governance may have. Franklyn Lisk draws from his experiences at the International Labour Organisation to conceptualise the role of the private sector within wider understandings of the theory and practice of tripartite partnerships. The paper considers how HIV/AIDS affects investment, business and enterprise, and the balance between the needs of private sector interests and labour. In so doing, Lisk teases out the achievements and potential for private sector inclusion within the HIV/AIDS response and the implications this has for processes of governance within the response.

The fourth section focuses on the governance of HIV/AIDS in regard to global governance and multisectoralism by focusing on the role of multisectorality in regards to two processes of international organisation support: the Global Fund to fight AIDS, Tuberculosis and Malaria, and the World Bank. Felicity Hatendi-Gutu's chapter, 'Institutional participation, accountability and transparency in the HIV/AIDS response', offers a nuanced perspective of the role of the state in relation to global governance and international organisation by focusing specifically upon the institutional collaboration between the state, the Global Fund and the UNDP. Of specific interest is the dichotomy between the Government of Zimbabwe's position within the international system and the willingness of the Global Fund to maintain and develop operations within this context. Particular to Hatendi-Gutu's chapter is the limitations experienced in terms of feedback and reciprocal accountability mechanisms between those in-country mechanisms of the Fund and recipients of Fund aid and the Global Fund in Geneva, and the implications this has for how we understand participation and accountability within the context of global governance. Sophie Harman's chapter focuses upon the role of the World Bank in harnessing and developing the concept of multisectoralism as a form of civil society and state participation within the Multi-Country AIDS Program (MAP) in Kenya, Tanzania and Uganda. Harman traces the origins of this form of engagement to the World Bank, pinpointing the linkages between global governance, national governance and civil society organisation engagement structures and the division of accountability therein. As such she argues for wider recognition of the role of the World Bank within the governance of the epidemic and the implications its involvement has for participation and accountability.

The book's central findings pertaining to participation and accountability are drawn together in the conclusion, which also highlights several further questions for discussion.

Part I

Role of the state and democratic governance in the HIV/AIDS response

1 AIDS, politics and governance

The impact of HIV/AIDS on the electoral process in Namibia, Malawi, Senegal, South Africa, Tanzania and Zambia

Kondwani Chirambo

Seeking knowledge on the impact of AIDS on democracy and governance in Africa has been at the core of social science for the past decade. Most of the empirical work in this field has tended to interrogate the socioeconomic implications of AIDS, however, presumably due to the availability of data. It is therefore barely five years since any serious attempts were made to unravel the political dynamics of the AIDS pandemic in Africa. According to the Joint United Nations Programme on HIV/AIDS (UNAIDS) estimates, between 33.4–46 million people worldwide are living with HIV (UNAIDS 2006). Sixty-three per cent of the cases (25.4 million) are in Sub-Saharan Africa (UNAIDS/WHO global reports 2004; 2006). HIV prevalence in Africa ranges from 0.7–9 per cent in countries such as Senegal in West Africa; one per cent in the North Africa region; to between 15–30 per cent in adult populations in most of Southern Africa – the region most affected by the epidemic (CHGA 2005; UNAIDS/WHO 2005).

Because the trends in mortality suggest that the relatively younger, and certainly the skilled and semi-skilled segment of the labour force are bearing the brunt of AIDS, these scenarios in turn have begun to generate a new wave of academic inquiry regarding the future of Africa's democracies: the unprecedented attrition of AIDS amongst the skilled labour force could possibly have severe effects on productivity, service delivery and subsequently citizen confidence in elected government if electioneering promises remained unfulfilled (Youde 2001; Mattes 2003: IDASA /HEARD/DARU Report 2002). The loss of elected leaders and professionals running political institutions such as parliament, political parties, electoral systems, electoral management bodies, judicial systems, finance ministries among others, was expected to undermine the mechanics of decision-making, institutional sustainability and effectiveness (Chirambo and Caesar 2003). Schonteich (2003) assumed that the higher incidences of orphaning would also increase crime and contribute to policing headaches in countries such as South Africa. In addition, it was posited that a disgruntled and largely unhealthy citizenry would likely rebel against the state, or withdraw from political life – a general weakening of social cohesion in the long term was envisaged (Mattes 2003).

While the Institute for Democracy in South Africa (IDASA) has investigated some of these phenomena, its ambition was to map areas of the political landscape that would effectively demonstrate the impact of, and also provide a basis for, targeted strategies against AIDS. IDASA's research was designed at a time when much of the region that comprises the Southern African Development Community (SADC)[1] was involved in protracted discussions on electoral reform to deepen democracy amongst its members. Several countries in the region had already been engaged in national debates on changing electoral models that were largely inherited from colonialism. These debates on reform have been motivated by many factors, some of which are attributed to opposition demands for fair representation, gender balance and ethnic diversity. Except for Lesotho, where the electoral system was changed following post-election conflict in 1998, none of the other SADC countries have concluded talks, presumably due to the reluctance of incumbents who view these changes as potentially denuding their authority (Chirambo 2008: 8). Elections, a defining feature of modern democracies, can evidently be undermined by many factors, including corruption, and unfairly unequal access to resources and communication systems. The significance of AIDS in this equation is only beginning to be understood and appreciated by some of the influential regional bodies involved in electoral processes such as the SADC Parliamentary Forum. In what ways therefore, one might ask, does AIDS impact on the electoral process? What are the governance implications of these impacts? How should governments respond, if there are any impacts at all?

Hypothesis and conceptual frameworks

This paper presents the findings of studies conducted between 2003 and 2007, which attempt to respond to these and other related concerns. The studies covered Namibia, Malawi, Tanzania, South Africa, Senegal and Zambia. They also make reference to Lesotho and Zimbabwe in respect of the electoral system. IDASA chose the countries based on the HIV prevalence rates and the electoral model in order to achieve comparability. The central analytical concept, operationalised through a focus on the *electoral process*, is *democratic governance* with particular regard to the notions of *participation* and *accountability*. The main hypothesis is that the impact of HIV/AIDS undermines the electoral process. The electoral process as defined in this study is characterised by rules, institutions and a set of political actors. Because of the significance of the electoral system to the political trajectory of the modern state, this paper will dedicate itself largely to relating to this institution. The first part of this paper presents the problems and key findings of the research. The second section engages in more depth with these findings, their implications and recommendations.

The project responds to the question: What is the impact of HIV/AIDS on the electoral process in Africa? To explore the question, the project has investigated the following areas of the electoral process:

- Electoral systems: Increased deaths amongst elected representatives will be financially demanding on the state as by-elections mount in countries employing simple member majority (SMM) systems and mixed member proportional (MMP) systems. These electoral models may in time be rendered unsustainable
- Parliamentary configuration: Weaker political parties will likely lose policy influence as they fail to recapture seats that are declared vacant following deaths amongst their elected representatives. By-elections will likely favour parties with the most resources
- Electoral management and administration: The management of the voters' roll will be problematic because of too many dead voters might overburden institutions that do not employ modern technology. The loss of skilled and support personnel employed by the electoral management boards (EMBs) might affect service delivery
- Political parties: Succession, finances and support bases may all be affected by attrition to AIDS amongst cadres, leaders and stalwarts. This might weaken viable opposition over time.
- Voter and civic participation: People infected and affected by HIV/AIDS will withdraw from elections due to lack of enthusiasm, the impact of sickness, stigma and discrimination.

All the five areas of focus have some influence on the nature and quality of governance. Of these, the electoral system will be paramount in the configuration of power. Electoral systems are the institutional devices that translate votes cast into seats in parliament. Depending on the model adopted by a particular country, electoral systems can maximize diversity in governance and afford marginalised sections of society opportunities to contribute to the setting of national priorities, including AIDS polices. While elections may be understood as the process through which citizens choose their leaders by casting ballots; electoral systems are explained here as the method or formula that translates the votes cast into seats in parliament (Matlosa *et al.* 2007).

Parliament, therefore, is the outcome of the operationalisation of electoral systems and elections. Oversight on government conduct is essential to the functioning of a democracy, and in many ways a representative parliament should be able to deliberate and enact laws that positively affect the welfare of the majority of the people. The relative independence of the electoral commission as defined in the legal and constitutional framework, and the integrity of its commissioners and professional staff, will also have a profound effect on how the outcomes of the poll are perceived. In the context of the AIDS pandemic, we would view the electoral management body as the institution that must institute measures to ensure that disadvantaged persons, including the infirm, pregnant women, and among others, people living with HIV/AIDS (PLWHAs), are able to vote without hindrance. Given the large numbers of citizens across Africa who are either infected with, or affected by, HIV/AIDS, facilitating reasonable access to the poll might have significant value in terms of levels of participation and, consequently, the legitimacy of the winners.

The political impact of the electoral system

Researchers on electoral systems underline the pivotal role these institutions play in influencing the future of a nation. Made up of laws and rules, the electoral system has been found to be critical to the configuration of power in governance structures and therefore influencing who decides on national priorities (Reynolds *et al.* 2005). The electoral system, in this regard, is one of the key institutional devices that facilitate participation of citizens in selecting policy options that would potentially improve their welfare and, more specifically, their access to life-sustaining opportunities of education, employment and health.

Electoral system types

There are four electoral systems that have been compared by IDASA in respect of the AIDS pandemic. For the purposes of this discussion, however, we shall focus mainly on three electoral system types – first-past-the-post (FPTP), proportional representation (PR) and MMP – and compare how they may be affected by HIV/AIDS.

Single member plurality or first-past-the-post

The FPTP system is defined by small voting districts or constituencies. The country is demarcated into electoral zones (constituencies) and political parties field one candidate each to compete for the constituency seat. Independent candidates can compete as well in most cases. The candidate who receives the most votes is declared the winner. In FPTP, when the seat falls vacant, a new election or by-election is called and all registered political parties may compete for it all over again. This is regardless of whether the vacancy arises as a result of a parliamentary representative resigning from

Table 1.1

Countries	*Electoral system*
Tanzania	FPTP
Malawi	FPTP
Zambia	FPTP
Zimbabwe	FPTP
South Africa	PR
Lesotho	MMP
Senegal	Parallel

their party or by dying. Botswana, Malawi, Mauritius, Swaziland, Tanzania, Zambia and Zimbabwe employ this model, inherited from British colonialism. FPTP or SMP are relatively stronger on accountability, as leaders are directly elected by the voters and may lose power in succeeding polls if their performance is adjudged to be poor. Some of the main criticisms of this system include its tendency to lead to the marginalization of ethnic minorities. It is also weak in terms of promoting gender balance due to the difficulties women face in highly competitive patriarchal environments. The FPTP model usually leads to a de facto bi-party system.

The SMM system bears similarities to FPTP, in that the country may be divided into electoral constituencies. However, the SMM requires that the winner achieves an absolute majority of votes (over 50 per cent). Employed largely in presidential polls, the SMM will normally provide for a run-off if none of the candidates attains 51 per cent of the vote. In the SADC region, Angola has used this model for its presidential elections. The SMM's main advantage is its facilitation of a legitimate winner of elections.

Proportional representation

Although global trends suggest that the PR systems are gaining in popularity due to their supposed contribution to conflict resolution (Matlosa *et al.* 2007), they do have their critics. There are many varieties of PR, of which the list systems are most common. PR systems are defined by large voting districts with an entire country constituting the constituency, for instance. The competition is between political parties and the seats in parliament are allocated on the basis of the proportion of the national vote that each party gains. For example, a party that wins 65 per cent of the total votes casts will theoretically secure 65 per cent of the seats in parliament. The parties will appoint its representatives from a list submitted to the EMB prior to the election, usually with the names in the upper sections occupying the available slots first. Of the SADC countries, Angola, Mozambique, Namibia and South Africa use the PR model.

Unlike FPTP, which is often linked to a proliferation of political parties that lack policy focus and ideology, PR models are linked to the opposite effect. This is because political parties will need to have wide-ranging and broad-based policies to ensure they attract enough of the national vote to reach the minimum threshold to secure a presence in parliament. The PR model facilitates gender diversity as women can be deliberately infused into party lists for parliament. It is suitable for conflict resolution as minority parties will have an opportunity to gain a foothold in parliament, particularly when there is a low minimum threshold; in this model, because of the low thresholds, nearly every vote contributes to electing a candidate. Other advantages are:

- promotes nationwide campaigns as opposed to parties restricting themselves to (ethnic or traditional) strongholds;
- power-sharing between parties is possible; and

- greater stability and longevity of government. No recourse to by-elections is necessary when vacancies occur, and there is therefore no disruption to power configurations in parliament.

The PR system's weaknesses include:

- party coalitions can cause a paralysis of governance when no consensus is reached on critical national issues;
- it might provide opportunities for the presence in parliament of extremist parties; and
- citizens cannot hold elected leaders accountable because the political party retains the mandate to appoint MPs from its dedicated list. There is no public input into who goes onto the closed party list (Reynolds et al 2005; Matlosa *et al.* 2007).

Mixed systems

Although MMP and the parallel system are both categorised as 'mixed', they have distinct differences. The MMP, by implication, minimises the weaknesses of both PR, FPTP and other systems by combining them. The MMP system facilitates the election of one group of members of parliament (MPs) or councillors through FPTP, and the other through the PR system. In MMP any disproportionalities arising from the FPTP (or other system) is compensated for by the PR element. Only one SADC country has adopted the MMP system at national level thus far, namely Lesotho (EISA 2003). While employing PR for national elections, South Africa uses MMP for its local government polls.

The parallel system is also classified as mixed. These models use PR and FPTP (or other system), operating side by side. The main difference with the MMP, however, is that while in the former the PR component compensates for disproportional outcomes from FPTP (or other system), in the parallel model the two systems are independent of each other and are separately managed. Seychelles is the only country in the SADC region that uses the parallel system (Reynolds *et al.* 2005); of the six countries in the IDASA's studies, Senegal is the only country employing the model. While it is logical to assume that the mixed systems inherit both the strengths and weaknesses of PR and FPTP, more studies need to be undertaken in regard to how MPs view each other in terms of their legitimacy: would directly elected MPs see themselves as being the 'true' representatives of the people, for instance, given their clearly defined relationship with the voter?

The impact of AIDS on governance

Barnett and Whiteside (2002) describe AIDS as 'a long wave event', one that demands strategic visions to address the impacts on current and future generations. A review of literature on AIDS suggests the pandemic has social, economic and political dynamics (Poku *et al.* 2007). As a result of AIDS, life expectancy in Southern Africa has declined from 60 years to below 40 years in the most affected countries, particularly in the sub-region defined as the SADC. Although the SADC region constitutes less than two per cent of the global population, it accounts for approximately 39 per cent, or 14.9 million, of the 38.6 million people living with HIV (end 2006). The added burden of 41 per cent of all children orphaned by AIDS exacerbates the side-effects of this pandemic (SADC 2006).

In this regard, social scientists present some compelling arguments on why the path of the pandemic may, over time, compromise governance: the manner in which countries manage their political, economic and social affairs. The pandemic's unprecedented effects on the adult populations, particularly on the most skilled of these populations who fall within the highly vulnerable 15–49 age cohort, raised concerns about economic performance, food security, public service efficiency and social cohesion. These assertions have in some cases been supported by empirical evidence. For instance, agriculture, the mainstay of the SADC region, has been the most affected by the loss of experienced labour, according to the Food and Agricultural Organisation (FAO). FAO estimates that more than seven million workers were lost to the epidemic across all sectors. The SADC Secretariat, housed in Gaborone, Botswana, also acknowledges the pandemic's effect on business in the sub-region as productivity declines due to absenteeism and deaths amongst workers, and profit margins are undermined as spending on sickness and death benefits rises (SADC 2003).

Recent forecasts on Southern Africa suggest that the region will not be able to fulfil the Millennium Development Goal 6: halving and reversing the spread of HIV/AIDS (malaria and other major diseases) by 2015. Despite the fact that the number of people on antiretroviral therapy (ART) in low- and middle-income countries almost doubled in 2005 from 720,000 to 1.3 million, new infections exceeded this figure at 4.9 million in the same year (UN General Assembly 16th session 2006). The SADC region is also anticipated to fail to achieve Millennium Development Goal 1: redress extreme poverty and hunger, which is closely related to the management of HIV/AIDS. ART uptake requires good nutrition and yet food insecurity and child malnutrition remain likely to constitute relentless adversaries for the foreseeable future. Similarly, maternal health is experiencing regression due to the relatively high trends of mortality among mothers, which are being attributed mainly to HIV/AIDS. The multiple challenges of human development bearing down on the continent force Africans to confront a range of interlinked problems: disease, poverty, food insecurity, poor infrastructure, low literacy rates, etc.

Governance in the context of HIV/AIDS

Advocates of governance, particularly the normative notion of 'good' or democratic governance, as a framework for dealing with these multisectoral challenges posed by HIV/AIDS, are also quick to point to the elusive nature of the concept (UNDP 1997; UNDP 2002; Hyden *et al.* 2004). There has long been no consensus about what constitutes governance, and moreover what is meant by governance in the context of HIV/AIDS. Contemporary thinking suggests that governance encompasses values, policies and institutions that allow for interaction and collaboration between state and non-state actors in implementing development projects (UNDP 1997; Cheema 2000; UNDP 2000; UNDP 2002).

Some key constituent elements of democratic governance for which there is broader consensus include freedom of expression and association, vibrant civil societies, gender equity and equality, rule of law, fundamental human rights, media freedom and free and fair elections. These elements are deemed to encourage participation and mutual accountability, thereby increasing effectiveness in the implementation of policy. First, a democratic government will likely observe and uphold human rights or may be more sensitive to public opinion on matters of treatment, care and support to the AIDS sick than an autocratic regime (Mattes 2003). The case of the South African government and its concession to demands by civil for comprehensive and unfettered access to treatment for all is one such highlight. Second, governance democratised, or opened up to free contestation from the local tier, allows civil society to create a citizen-based agenda in the framing of policy and the monitoring of policy deliverables (De Wit 2000).

For a government to be considered effective and accountable, the decisions it takes must be the enforceable product of the will of the people. Governance is therefore not any good unless it particularly translates into sustainable human development (the expansion of life choices and opportunities that lead to improved literacy, employment and health, among other benefits) (UNDP/ZHDR 2000). In this regard, the decline in life expectancy to below 50 years in most of Southern Africa due to HIV/AIDS; and the epidemic's potential to catalyse institutional weakness justifies a response that mobilizes cross-sectoral support for efforts aimed at improving human welfare. Effective government in this regard could be evaluated based on human output measurements, such as the number of people receiving ART, antenatal care, primary health care and those who are in need of these services. The gap between the two is then taken as the measure of governmental effectiveness in providing for the health needs of its citizens (see, for example, Natrass 2008). It is through monitoring this gap, between a rights-based need and the actual delivery of these needed services, that elected officials, the locally elected officials most specifically, are held accountable. Expenditure on health, specifically on HIV/AIDS, provides another important measure of political commitment by governments to the epidemic. Budget tracking and analysis is often framed against international commitments that governments sign up to. The Abuja declaration of 2001, for example, commits member states of the African Union (AU) to devoting 15 per cent of the national budget to healthcare (Mukotsanjera 2008).

The political challenge that HIV/AIDS presents to the governance dynamic is much more subtle: The experienced officials, whom affected countries need desperately to deliver on their health and other needs, will themselves stand in the way of danger. Because they may be ill, they might not attend parliamentary debates on a regular basis; because they are stigmatised, they might be reluctant to interact in public places, affecting their effectiveness and accountability, and finally, because they succumb to mortality, their absence might stall certain development projects until suitable replacements are elected. This discussion therefore raises some fundamental questions, which will be the main focus of this chapter:

- What are the political and governance implications of rising deaths amongst elected representatives?
- In what ways does HIV/AIDS affect voting age populations who elect the officials to decide on governance priorities?
- Does the severity of HIV/AIDS necessitate institutional transformation in order to absorb the epidemic's impacts?

The following section discusses the findings of the IDASA studies, which in unravelling the impact of AIDS on the electoral process, also expands on this discussion on AIDS, politics and governance.

Findings

The proplems and impacts of AIDS on electoral systems

The outcomes of the study address the five main areas highlighted in the introduction of the paper: the electoral system, parliamentary configuration, political parties, electoral management and administration, and voter participation. The findings rely on inferences drawn from analysing trends in mortality among elected representatives and their age cohorts, and the sum of effects that this has on the three main electoral models in the SADC region. This is because records of the actual causes of deaths of elected representatives, as with any citizen, are treated as confidential. Comparisons are drawn between mortality trends in the pre-AIDS period and in the AIDS era. With the exception of Zambia, none of the other countries had data before 1990. In such cases, we still examine the number of vacancies attributed to deaths as opposed to resignations, dismissals or other factors. Finally, by aggregating the causes of by-elections in countries that employ the FPTP system, IDASA was able to draw conclusions as to whether there were significant increases in by-elections during the AIDS era as opposed to the period before. It is worth noting that, while the analyses do not conclusively attribute deaths to AIDS, they nevertheless help to draw deductions from the pattern of deaths and their correlation to trends in AIDS deaths in the national population. High mortality among relatively younger politicians (40–55) provides a strong basis to link the deaths that have been attributed officially to 'long' or 'short' illness to the influence of the pandemic. Similar reasoning is applied to the population of registered voters (18–49 year olds in this category are considered the relatively younger cohort).

Mortality amongst African parliamentarians

Trends in this study show relatively large numbers of parliamentary vacancies arising due to deaths from undisclosed illnesses amongst MPs in Malawi, Tanzania, Zambia and, to a lesser extent, South Africa.

Countries with severe AIDS epidemics show distinct patterns of high mortality in the 1990s – the period in which AIDS would have peaked. Tracking the number of by-elections attributed to deaths from natural causes clarifies the trend. For instance, in Zambia, while only 6.44 per cent of the 46 by-elections held between 1964 and 1984 (in the AIDS-free era) were caused by MPs succumbing to natural deaths, the numbers rose dramatically between 1985–2006, (the phase when AIDS peaked) – in that period, at least 60 per cent of the 146 by-elections held were due to disease-related deaths of incumbent MPs. In addition, between 2002 and 2007, a total of 243 ward by-elections were held at local government level, in Zambia.

In Malawi, it is noticeable that there is a steady increase in the number of legislators who have passed away since 1994. There are more deceased MPs between the 1994–96 period – the height of the AIDS pandemic – compared to the 1999–2004 period, in which 23 MPs died between 1994 and 1999 and

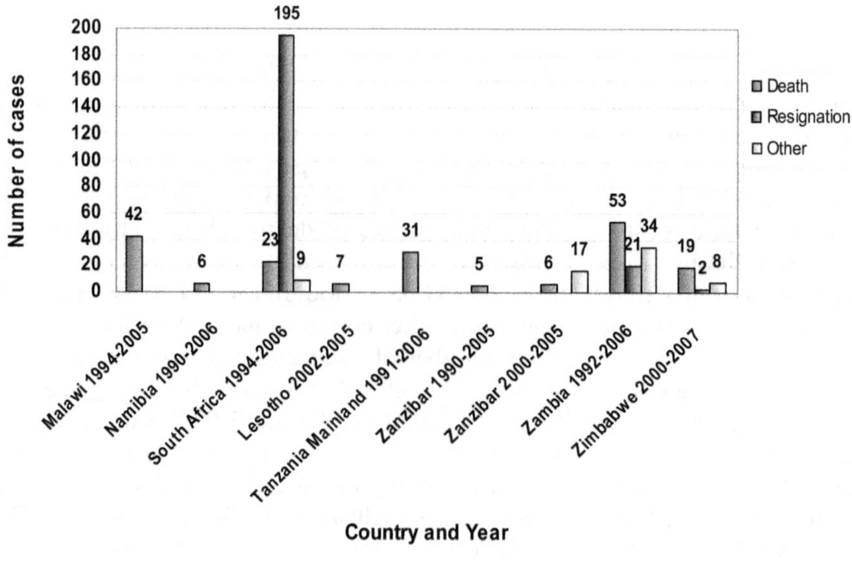

Figure 1.1
Source: Chirambo 2008.

12 between 1999 and 2004. A total of 42 MPs succumbed to mortality between 1994 and 2006. Out of a total of 193 MPs at the end of 2005, 87 (45 per cent) were below 50 years of age. If the causes were in any doubt, the speaker of the National Assembly of Malawi disclosed in the year 2000 that 28 MPs had died of HIV/AIDS-related complexes. Subsequent to his statement, Malawi lost seven MPs in a single year (2005). Tanzania has also experienced a rise in MP deaths between the early 1990s and 2006. According to official records, 31 MPs died between 1991 and 2006. Four deaths are attributed to car accidents and shootings, while the rest were caused by undisclosed 'long' and 'short' illnesses. Mortality at the House of Representatives in Zanzibar is relatively low, at five deaths in 1990–2005. The disparities between Zanzibar [less than 1 per cent prevalence and 4.7 per cent incidence in 2004 (UNAIDS/WHO 2005)], and Tanzania (7per cent HIV prevalence rate) mainland in terms of prevalence rates might be explained by the influence of religion or geographical position and size, among other things. Zanzibar, is predominantly Moslem, and is a much smaller geographical zone to cover with AIDS campaigns. While the influence of Islam needs further investigation, the case of Senegal, a predominantly Moslem state, where religious leaders used carefully crafted messages to deliver safe sex messages, might provide pointers to its potential. Religious leaders in Senegal apparently advised people who could not abstain to use condoms, an uncharacteristic position for clerics. In addition, the culture of dialogue is highlighted as one of the main reasons that led to effective networking amongst various interests in order to stem the spread of AIDS in Senegal (Chirambo 2008: 21).

Zimbabwe has held a series of 29 by-elections between 2000 and 2005. Nineteen of these were caused by the deaths of MPs to undisclosed illnesses.

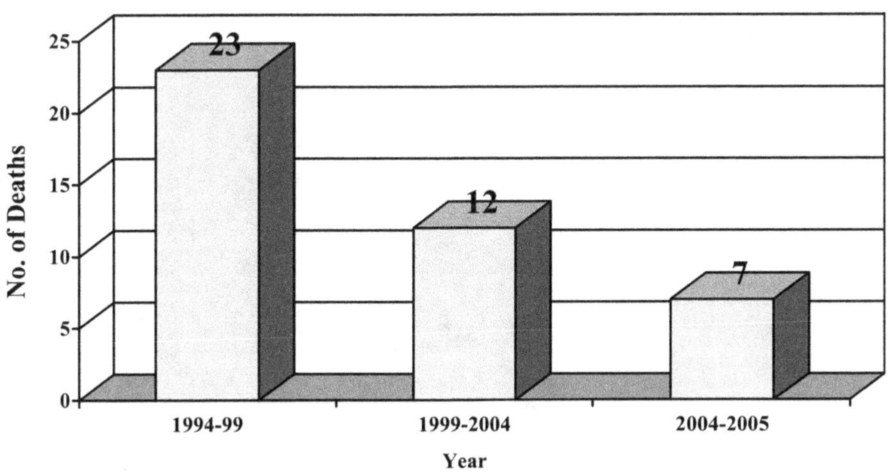

Figure 1.2
Source: Chirambo 2008.

At least one vacancy was caused by resignation of an MP on account of ill health, and another was appointed to higher office. Additional causes for the vacancies in official records show that at least one MP was dismissed. Six constituencies – Buhera North, Hurungwe East, Mutoko South, Chiredzi North, Gokwe North and Gokwe South – had their results nullified by the high court following petitions by losing candidates.

Impact of AIDS in countries with PR and MMP

As the national prevalence rate ranges between 0.7 and 9 per cent (UNAIDS 2006), it may not be surprising that Senegal in the 1990s only recorded three deaths amongst MPs in 2001–6. Namibia, on the Southwest coast of Africa, recorded 6 deaths among MPs from the between 1990 and 2006. Four of these were from the National Assembly and two from the National Council. Information released to the public through the media attributed the deaths to diabetes, vehicle accident, long and short illnesses, and heart attack. Overall, the death rates among the 98 elected members of both houses have remained comparatively low. As in South Africa, the PR system employed at national level is relatively cheaper to manage than FPTP would be when vacancies occur as no by-elections are required.

South Africa's 400-member parliament has had a high turnover for a variety of reasons. Official records show that 227 MPs departed (resigned, appointed to higher positions or dismissed) between 1994 and 2006. Twenty-three of the

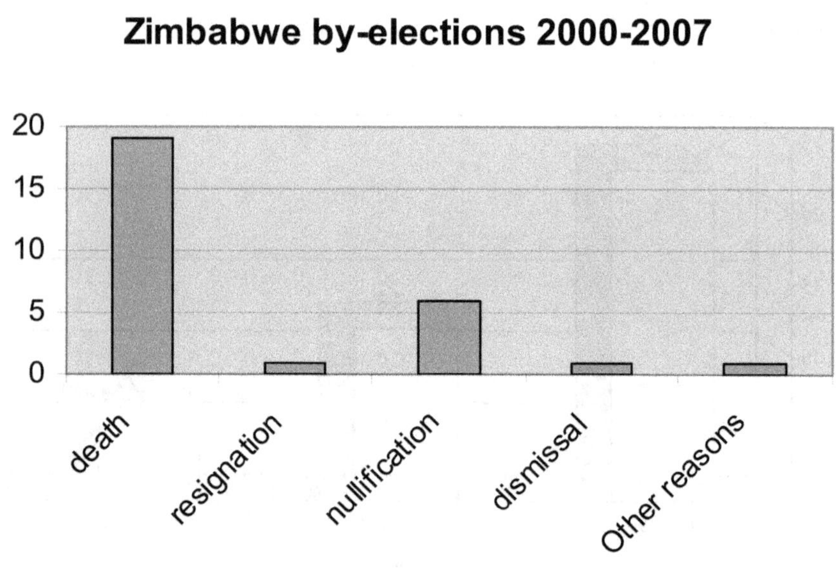

Figure 1.3
Source: Zesn/Chirambo 2008.

vacancies were caused by the deaths of MPs, the causes of which were not released. The information made available by the South African parliament on mortality covered only the post-apartheid era, which covers a relatively short time span. Because South Africa uses the PR system, the replacement of MPs is not subject to by-elections and does not require public voting. This renders the PR more cost-effective than the majoritarian systems, but it must be remembered that while South Africa appears insulated from the financial costs of replacing deceased leaders at national level, it also holds by-elections at a local level to replace directly elected councillors under the MMP system. In 2001, a total of 79 by-elections were held. Of these, 27 were in KwaZulu-Natal and nine in Gauteng. Michael Sachs (2002) research of 2001 indicates that of the 79 by-elections in 2001, 34 were caused by a councillor's resignation from his or her post, 33 were caused by the death of a councillor and 12 resulted from the expulsion of a councillor either from the party or the council concerned. The MMP's vulnerability is further demonstrated by Lesotho, where by-elections have had to be held to replace MPs who are elected through the FPTP stream. Eight by-elections were held in 2002–5, the period in which the modified MMP electoral model was instituted.

Average ages of MPs and vulnerability factors

The information made available to this project suggests that the parliaments under review are manned by MPs who may be regarded as being in the vulnerable age groups. The current Zambian parliament, elected in 2006, and with an average age of 46, is the youngest, followed by Namibia and Malawi at 51 years; Tanzania has a relatively higher average of 54, while South Africa and Senegal come in at 55 years. The growth of multiparty politics could be a major contributing factor to the introduction of relatively younger politicians in national parliaments in the past 15 years.

Implications of MP mortality

Frequent deaths amongst elected leaders have a number of governance implications. First, it causes the affected constituencies to lose voice in parliament. In the majority systems, MPs are expected to be the fundamental link to the communities, more so than the local councillor, perhaps given the higher profile of the former. Communities will call on their MP for both developmental and personal needs, including assistance toward funeral costs. In countries such as Malawi and Tanzania, constituency leadership posts have remained vacant for long periods. On the Tanzania mainland, six constituencies – Kisesa, Mbeya Vijijini, Ulanga Mashariki, Kasulu Mashariki, Rahaleo and Kilombero – had no MPs by the December 2005 general elections. Their MPs had died during the 2000–2005 parliamentary sitting. During the 1995–2000 parliaments, ten MPs died. By-elections in Malawi were delayed for up to one year after the 2004 national elections. The Electoral Commission attributed

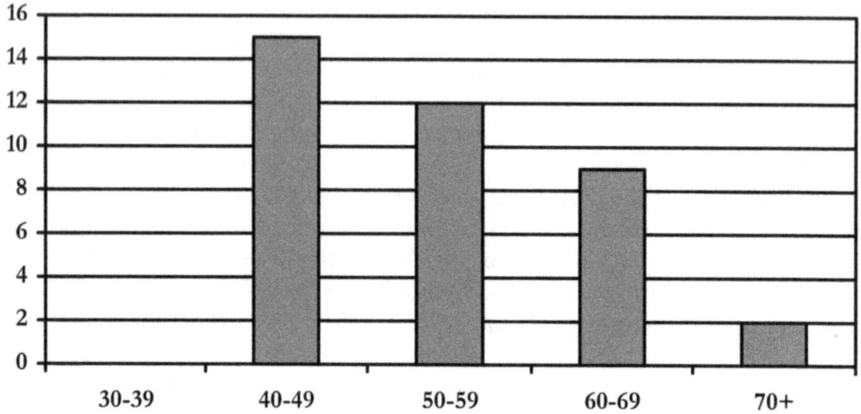

Figre 1.4 Age cohort and numbers of deceased MPs 1990–2003 Zambia

the delay to lack of finances. Lack of financial resources also caused the government to indefinitely postpone local government elections. There are other priorities, such as food security and debt relief, that take precedence in one of the world's poorest countries and the government decided to forego the demands of electoral democracy. This occurrence, by itself, will perhaps underline the issue of electoral sustainability: in the age of AIDS, when by-elections occur in rapid succession at both national and local levels, can resource-stressed countries sustain majoritarian electoral models? With treatment, understandably, the rates of deaths will slow down, but the costs will remain onerous regardless, for each death.

Second, numerous by-elections will likely attract fewer people to vote. Certainly, trends in by-elections revealed in Sachs (2002) illustrate lower levels of participation in local by-elections in South Africa compared with national polls. By-elections require significant investments by the state, political parties and election monitors. Large-scale public education campaigns have to be mounted each time, with considerable resources used for media messages, discussions, and printing of posters and fresh ballots. The organisational nightmares, coupled with contending priorities on the part of the voter, will conspire to reduce participation and impact on the legitimacy of the winner.

Changing power configurations in national parliaments

Numerous by-elections inadvertently affect the smaller political parties more, because of their lack of financial and organisational pedigree. In this study, Zambia and Zimbabwe provide examples of situations where relatively strong opposition parties have experienced parliamentary decline due to their failure to recapture seats that fall vacant or to claim additional slots through by-elections. In the 2000 Zimbabwean parliamentary elections, the Zimbabwe African National Union-Patriotic Front (ZANU-PF) won 62 seats of the 120 available, while the opposition Movement for Democratic Change (MDC) secured 57. A lone seat went to the other opposition ZANU-Ndonga party. The country held 14 by-elections in the first four years following the 2000 legislative polls. Eight of the by-elections were caused by the deaths of parliamentary representatives to undisclosed illnesses. Through victories in most by-elections, ZANU-PF had increased its parliamentary strength from 62 to 67 seats by 2004. It had succeeded in securing five extra seats from the MDC whose portfolio shrank within the same period from 57 to 52 seats.

In Zambia, the ruling Movement for Multi-party Democracy (MMD) increased their vote from 46 per cent to 54 per cent representation in parliament between the 2001 and 2006 presidential and parliamentary general elections. MMD's toughest opponents, the United Party for National Development (UPND) and the United National Independence Party (UNIP), slipped from 49 to 43per cent and 8.7 to 6per cent parliamentary representations respectively. Since elections in both countries are highly competitive, marginal advantages might have significant impacts on how priorities are set. Certainly in the case of Zimbabwe, the socioeconomic crisis currently rocking the country will relegate matters such AIDS to the backseat because the current regime is preoccupied with political survival above all else.

Economic costs of replacing deceased MPs through by-elections

Majoritarian systems are costly to maintain both in both political and economic terms. AIDS accelerates the rate at which vacancies occur. As stated, the combined effect of resignations, dismissals and deaths will increase the regularity of elections and therefore the economic and human resources required to sustain the system in its current form. In December 2005, the six by-elections in Malawi cost an estimated MK65 million ($US474,799.12), which translated into approximately MK10.8 million ($US78,889.70) per constituency. Zambia's by-elections cost US$235,849 on average. Tanzania's by-elections cost US$416,000 on average. From the experience of Lesotho, the MMP is not insulated from costs: the seven by-elections held in Lesotho since the country modified the electoral model in 2002 from FPTP to an MMP system, each cost approximately R1 million (US$143,601). At the local level, the cumulative effect of holding too many local by-elections in South Africa's MMP system might have a significant bearing on national resources in due course as well. A ward poll can cost approximately R30,000.00 (US$4,000 at the rand rate to the US dollar at the time of publishing).

Voter mortality and the voter register

Except for Namibia, all the SADC countries covered in this study employ public service workers as election officers to compliment their permanent staff during elections. Most are openly acknowledging the devastating effect that the loss of public workers, particularly teachers, is having on their ability to retain experience and capacity. Approximately 200,000 of Sub-Saharan Africa's 650,000 teachers are projected to die of AIDS (Chirambo: 2008). While the actual impact in terms of capacity of EMBs has not been quantified due to lack of reliable data, the challenges of managing voter rolls has been the more apparent complication that arises from increased AIDS deaths amongst electorates. In order to gauge the distinct challenges AIDS may pose for EMBs, we compare Malawi with South Africa.

Malawi, a country grappling with the installation of a credible citizen, voter and death registration system, provides the most compelling case. The country still operates a colonial death registration system whereby local chiefs are entrusted with reporting all deceased subjects to the local authorities. It is an inherently low-efficiency mechanism and, by the admission of senior electoral officers, poses problems for government and the electoral commission in as far as purging the voter registers of dead citizens is concerned. The unreliability of the roll contributes to the lack of legitimacy that the current administration of President Bingu Wa Mutharika experiences. For instance, in the 1999 general elections, the Malawi Electoral Commission registered 5,071,822 voters. The Malawi Electoral Commission (MEC) claimed to have removed 106,086 registered voters from the roll in the five years prior to the 2004 general elections. The figure of 6,668,839 registered voters was announced for the 18 May 2004 presidential and parliamentary elections, which was highly contentious. On the contrary, the National Statistics Office (NSO)'s projections during the same period suggested that 5,594,081 people aged 18 years or older were eligible to vote in Malawi. The MEC failed to explain where the excess of one million voters emanated from.

South Africa, on the other hand, has the most technologically advanced system of all the countries under review. It uses bar-coded identity cards (IDs) with electronic compatibility between citizen and voter registers. South Africa purges dead voters on a monthly basis. Based on this data set, it was established in the South Africa study that 1,488,242 of the country's registered voters died between 1999 and 2003 out of a total of 20,674,926 people who were on the voters' roll for the 2004 general elections. Deaths are

Table 1.2

Country	*Electoral system*	*Average cost of by-elections*
Tanzania Mainland	FPTP	US$ 416,000
Zanzibar	FPTP	US$ 45,000
Zambia	FPTP	US$ 235,849
Malawi	FPTP	US$ 78,000
Lesotho	MMP	US$ 143 601

Compiled by Idasa.
Using the rate of 1 USD= 6.9637 rand, September 25th 2007.

concentrated in the 20–49 years and 60–79 age groups. IDASA argues that the sharp increases in mortality – in some cases up to 200 per cent – among registered voters between the ages of 20–49, particularly among women in the 30–39 age bracket can, to a large extent, be explained by AIDS.

The data shows a strong correspondence between the profiles that IDASA's analysis generates and those that have been described by the expert demographers in the field of HIV/AIDS.

Stigma and discrimination as impediments to citizen participation in politics

It is noted in an IDASA study that there are silent exclusionary practices in the political elites who have taken to marginalising fellow aspirants to elective office at the remotest sign of illness. This was especially evident in Zambia, where prospective candidates accused their opponents of being HIV positive. As many citizens have yet to come to terms with living with HIV/AIDS, the implication is that such candidates are unlikely to be elected. Political party leaders interviewed in the study indicated their reluctance to adopt PLWHAs in their ranks because they were viewed as 'a potential by-election'. While politicians in Namibia, Malawi, Tanzania, South Africa and Senegal were less forthright about embracing PLWHAs into party systems, they all converged on the same plane when it came to disclosure of their HIV status. The mantra is that disclosure is politically costly, since no political party or member of the public would entertain somebody who was seen as on the verge of death. We can interpret this another way: because politics are usually

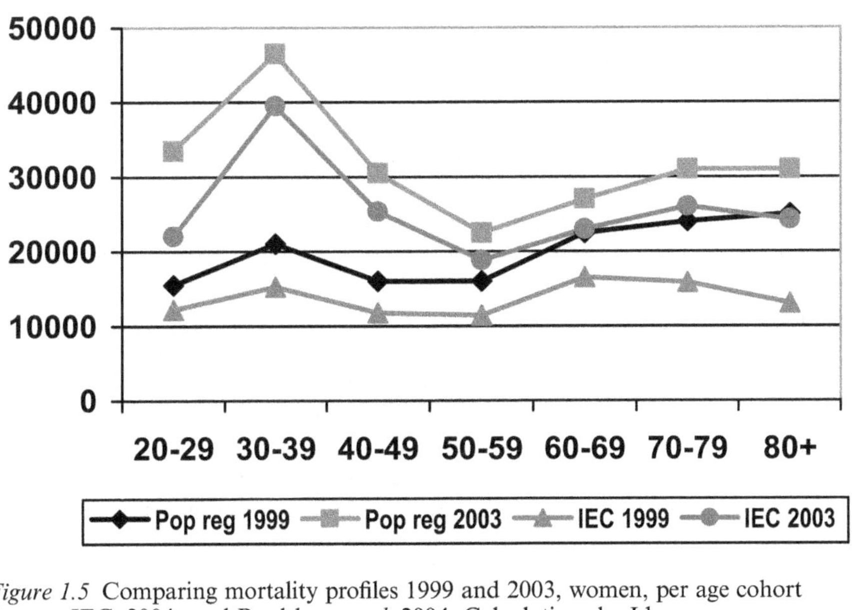

Figure 1.5 Comparing mortality profiles 1999 and 2003, women, per age cohort
Source: IEC, 2004e and Bradshaw *et al.* 2004. Calculations by Idasa.

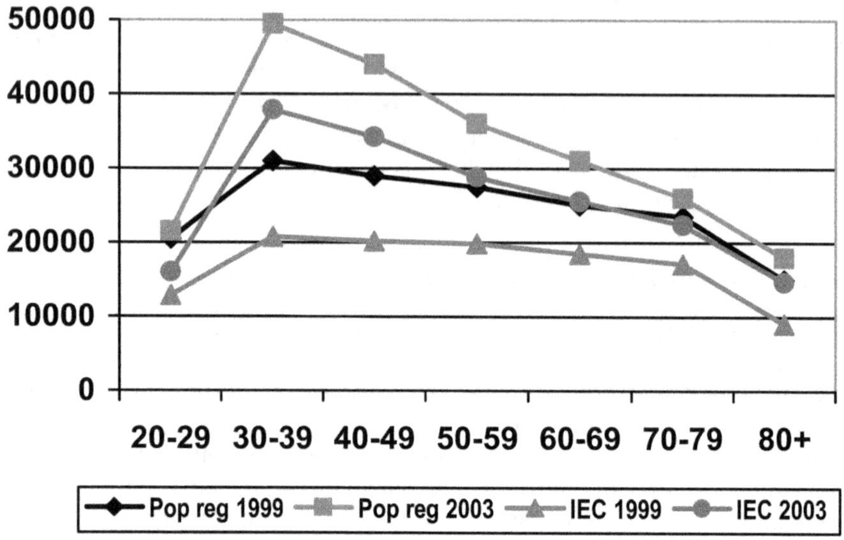

Figure 1.6 Comparing mortality profiles 1999 and 2003, men, per age cohort
Source: IEC, 2004e and Bradshaw *et al.* 2004. Calculations by Idasa.

the only means of livelihood for those in power in the developing world, the loss of political office could translate into the loss of significant economic benefits as well. These considerations may have contributed to the highly improbable record of non-disclosure amongst senior elected officials in government and parliamentary structures. To date, no elected official is on record as carrying HIV. At the grassroots levels, it is observed that AIDS sickness may prevent voters from participation in elections because of the physical demands of queuing and walking to polling stations, the absence of ablution facilities, and the fear of discrimination, among other things.

Although the levels of stigma and discrimination differ from country to country, it was only in South Africa that PLWHAs in Kwazulu Natal expressed fears that fellow voters might be violent against them. Historically, South Africa has documented a number of cases where PLWHAs have been assaulted, the worst being the stoning to death of Gugu Dlamini in 1998 (Fredriksson and Kanabus 2004). The opinions from focus group discussions with PLWHAs and care givers are corroborated by the findings of studies on stigma and discrimination, particularly the South African Department of Health study (DoH 2003): that HIV/AIDS remains a taboo topic among some South African communities, especially in the rural enclaves. The sense of stigma, it seems, is strongest where people are symptomatic. Registered voters who were HIV positive said that most members of the communities would not stand in the same queue with someone with visible signs of disease, e.g. body rashes or sores (Chirambo 2006).

Conclusion

This discussion, though limited in its scope to the electoral arena, nevertheless provides a basis for us to begin to understand in what ways the pandemic interacts with political governance. The report does not measure the impact of AIDS on politics and governance, but rather discusses its findings within the said contexts. Measurement will require an examination of attendance records to evaluate the relationship between absenteeism by MPs and AIDS illness. It will call for an examination of records of the records of parliamentary proceedings to determine how MPs afflicted by HIV/AIDS may have become less effective in policy discussions; this might in turn require a level of openness by parliament, families of the deceased and communities in order to assess contributions or lack thereof by infected representatives over time.

By tracking deaths amongst MPs using by-elections, it has been possible to do two things: (i) establish a trend in deaths, the age cohorts of deceased persons; and (ii) establish the costs of replacing the deceased through fresh elections.

These approaches facilitate an informed discussion on the likelihood of HIV/AIDS causing institutional weakness. In this regard, the first impression is that the PR system is the most cost-effective model in the era of HIV/AIDS. The FPTP is certainly the most vulnerable in its current structure; MMP provides some insulation, but only to a limited extent.

We have noted the unusual pattern of deaths amongst elected leaders, particularly in the mid-1990s – a period when there was little or no access to ART for most Africans and when AIDS had peaked in the SADC region. We notice that the main cause of parliamentary vacancies is deaths to natural causes (undisclosed illnesses) in nearly all of the SADC countries in the study. The parliaments of the countries under investigation have MPs who can be described as falling within the vulnerable categories (sexually active groups in the 24–50 age range). In the case of Zambia, comprehensive data from 1964 to 2006 demonstrates a mortality profile that more clearly mimics the AIDS patterns in the general population. Senegal, a low prevalence country, shows no significant deaths amongst MPs. At one level, we note that frequent deaths amongst MPs tend to change the parliamentary power configurations in countries that use the FPTP electoral model. This extends the advantage to political parties with the most resources, which will often be in a much stronger position to compete in each by-election. Consequently, such parties may achieve two-third majority statuses allowing them great leverage over policy matters, even in cases where they may not have fared well at general elections. The importance of a two-third majority is not be underestimated, as it implies that the party in power will likely be able to pass crucial governance decisions without critical reference to the opposition. In the event that the parties that benefit from these by-elections have only a marginal interest in the long-term effects of AIDS on society, there may be serious repercussions to the human development aspirations of the most affected social groups.

The question of gender balance also arises. If the majority of deceased MPs are women, it is highly unlikely that political parties will find competitive female candidates to effectively contest the vacant portfolios in male-dominated societies. FPTP countries will therefore experience a decline in female representation despite efforts to achieve parity. At another level, we may raise concerns about the loss of seniority and experience in strategic governance institutions such as parliament. Political careers and pedigrees are built over generations; the loss of leaders below the ages of 65 in relatively large numbers would likely have some implications for the quality of governance.

The increase in deaths amongst MPs in Malawi, Tanzania, Zambia and Zimbabwe also highlights the issue of representation – or lack thereof. One of the key elements in governance is the participation of all marginalised citizens in decisions that affect their lives. What happens to constituencies that stay without MPs for extended periods of time? At a micro level, the loss of MPs, often viewed as champions of development by their constituencies, is certain to disadvantage the affected community in terms of their effective representation. Put simply, no one person performs exactly the same as another, so the loss of a representative might compromise participation in the political public sphere for the marginalised.

We also notice that large numbers of voters have died, with the younger 30–39 age cohort constituting the majority in South Africa. Comprehensive data is not available from the other five countries due to either the absence of institutionalised voter registration systems or migration to new systems in the recent past. In South Africa, however, because of a highly sophisticated citizen and voter registration system, we are able to analyse and correlate the voter mortality profile with deaths as a result of AIDS in the general population. The loss of voters might have the effect of reducing the pool of people available to participate in elections.

The above presents, in my view, compelling arguments for modifications of the FPTP system, particularly for countries that are already economically weak. I noted earlier that Malawi and Zambia's reliance on donor support, for instance, for some of their general elections is indicative of their inability to fully sustain the costs of managing an electoral process. The costs associated with holding by-elections, coupled with the desire by stakeholders within these countries to achieve diversity and representation in governance mechanisms, should provide a strong basis for reasoned action in terms of electoral reforms. Comprehensive reforms require a shift from current FPTP models to either PR or MMP. However, the experience of the last two decades shows that there are many interests at play in regard to electoral reforms, and a complete migration is unlikely to happen overnight unless there is a revolution. It is therefore more realistic to recommend that countries consider eliminating the requirement for by-elections and thereby allow the affected political parties to appoint replacement, without recourse to costly polls. This will also ensure that modifications to the electoral model do not compromise accountability, the factor for which the FPTP is profoundly known to be the stronger. To avoid weakening the accountability of modified FPTP systems, there could therefore be additional consideration to commit representatives to quarterly meetings with their constituencies. In South Africa councillors are required to do so in terms of the Municipal Systems Act of 2000 in Schedule 1 on the code of conduct. AIDS could be one of the key performance benchmarks for representatives in this regard.

The research also suggested that stigma and discrimination is rife amongst the political elite, and fear of ostracism from party ranks appears to explain the lack of openness. This phenomenon calls for innovative approaches to deal with it. It will be easier for countries using the PR system to scale this hurdle. One of the suggestions would be for countries such as South Africa to take the lead by encouraging political parties to appoint person(s) living openly with HIV/AIDS to the PR lists for forthcoming general elections, thereby deliberately infusing PLWHAs into the governance structures. Lesotho, with its MMP system, might also succeed with this proposition. It is more difficult for the FPTP countries, given the stigma and discrimination that still permeates society: the odds of a PLWHA winning a competitive election might not be that high. However, FPTP countries could exploit the seats for nominated MPs that are filled by presidential prerogative. In Zambia, eight of the 158 seats are for nominated members. Dominant parties, such as the MMD and the Botswana Democratic Party (BDP) in Botswana – which are not in immediate threat of losing an election – present the best prospect for change in this regard. An intervention of this nature would likely have huge impacts on negative perceptions of PLWHAs within society, in that it would be seen to normalise a condition often regarded as a death sentence or a plague.

Regular medical check-ups for MPs are essential, so that early interventions by doctors could be instituted. These might not necessarily entail HIV tests, but could be useful in identifying signs of deteriorating health or symptoms of HIV amongst elected officials. Workplace policies with strong, all-encompassing information, education and communication strategies need to be instituted to assist in developing pools of AIDS-competent MPs. Training and knowledge-building for parliamentarians to enable them to act on the political, social and economic challenges faced by constituencies and employ that knowledge in their oversight functions. There is, therefore, a need to identify champions in parliamentary bodies who would form the core of strategic parliamentary interventions.

The research further suggests that there are roles for the EMBs in the HIV/AIDS field. The impact of stigma and discrimination on participation, though only indicative in rural South Africa, deserves attention as it may be more extensive than this study suggests, with ramifications for the involvement of individuals infected with, and affected by, HIV/AIDS in politics. It is only when we increase the participation of PLWHAs and activists in policy processes that we can expect any significant levels of accountability on HIV/AIDS to enter the electoral arena. EMBs could assist by incorporating antidiscrimination messages in their voter education campaigns, which encourage more people to participate in elections and ensure there is tolerance to a greater degree of people who are ill. The Zanzibar Electoral Commission, for example, encouraged political parties to deploy AIDS awareness messages during the 2005 election in Tanzania.[2] Setting up special voting mechanisms for the disadvantaged might also be a consideration, for instance in South Africa. Such facilities should not be exclusively tailored to PLWHAs, to avoid accentuating stigma and discrimination; they should rather seek to engage all persons with disabilities and those challenged by ill health, among others. African countries will also need to upgrade their citizen and voter registration systems to ensure that the true size of registered voter populations is publicly known and the possibility of fraud is minimised or eliminated.

All these measures might contribute to increased participation and accountability, improving the citizens' capacity to make informed decisions on their choice of HIV/AIDS policy.

Notes

1 The SADC countries are: Angola, Botswana, the Democratic Republic of Congo (DRC), Lesotho, Mauritius, Malawi, Mozambique, Namibia, Seychelles, South Africa, Swaziland, Tanzania, Zambia and Zimbabwe.

2 Zanzibar and Tanganyika form one state under the Union of the Republic of Tanzania

Bibliography

Barnet T. (2007). HIV/AIDS, a long Wave Event: Sundering the Intergenerational Bond. In Poku N., Whiteside A., and Sandkjaer B. (eds) (2007). *AIDS and Governance.* England: Ashgate.

Bradshaw, D., Laubscher, R., Dorrington, R., Bourne, D., Timaeus, I. (2004). 'Unabated Rise in Number of Adult Deaths in South Africa', *South African Medical Journal*, April.

Brown, S., and Morton, B. (2008). *Reforming aid and development cooperation: Accra, Doha and beyond North-South Policy Institute* http://www.nsi-ins.ca/english/pdf/DAW_policy.pdf retrieved September 26, 2008

Caesar-Katsenga M., & Myburg M. (eds) (2006). *Parliament, Politics and AIDS.* Cape Town: Idasa

Cheema, G.S. (2000). *In Good Governance: A path to Poverty Eradication.* New York: United Nations Development Programme (UNDP).

Chirambo K., Erasmus C., and Nel N. (2003). Zambia Presidential, Parliamentary and Local Government Elections 2001. Evaluation of Donor Investments. Pretoria: Idasa

Chirambo, K., and Caesar, M. (eds) 2003. *AIDS and Governance in Southern Africa: Emerging Theories and Perspectives.* Pretoria: Idasa.

Chirambo, K. (2006). *Democratisation in the Age of HIV/AIDS; Understanding the Political Implications.* Cape Town: IDASA

Chirambo, K. (ed.) (2008). *The Political Cost of AIDS in Africa.* Cape Town: Idasa

Chipika J. T. (2007). *Current Macroeconomic Frameworks, Challenges and alternatives for the attainment of the Millennium Development Goals.* http://www.sarpn.org.za/document/d0002654/index.php

CHGA (2004). *Q & A on HIV/AIDS and Governance in Africa.* Addis Ababa: Commission for HIV/AIDS Governance in Africa/Economic Commission for Africa.

Department of Health (DoH) (2003). National HIV and Syphyllis Antenatal Seroprevalence Survey in South Africa. Summary Report. Pretoria.

De Wit, J. (2000). Towards Good Governance At The Local Level; The Role Of Grassroots Institutions. http://biblio.iss.nl/opac/uploads/wp/wp325.pdf, retrieved September 26, 2008

DPRU Policy Brief No. 01/p13, May 2001, Human Development Indicators in the SADC Region. University of Cape Town

EISA (2003). *Principles for Election Management, Monitoring and Observation in the SADC Region.* Johannesburg: Electoral Commissions Forum/EISA.

Fredriksson, J. and Kanabus, A. (eds) 2004. *HIV & AIDS Stigma and Discrimination: Attitudes towards HIV and AIDS.* http://www.avert.org/aidstigma.htm

Hyden G., Court J. & Mease K. (2004). *Making Sense of Governance: Empirical Evidence from 16 Countries.* London: Rienner.

IDASA/HEARD/DARU (2002). AIDS and Democracy Workshop for Researchers Report.

Matlosa K., Chiroro B., and Letsholo S. (2007). Politics of Electoral System Reform and Democratisation: Contemporary Trends in Southern Africa. EISA; Johannesburg. Conference paper.

Mattes, R. (2003). "Healthy Democracies? Potential Impact of HIV/AIDS on Democracy in Southern Africa", in Chirambo, K. and Caesar, M. (eds) *AIDS and Governance in Southern Africa: Emerging Theories and Perspectives.* Cape Town: Idasa.

Mukotsanjera V. (ed.) (2008). *HIV/AIDS Financing and Spending in Eastern and Southern Africa.* Cape Town: Idasa

Natrass, N. (2008). Are country reputations for good and bad leadership on AIDS deserved?: an exploratory quantitative analysis. *Journal of Public Health.* September

Poku N., Whiteside A. & Sandjaer B. (eds) (2007). AIDS and Governance: Ashgate: Hampshire.

Reynolds, A., Reilly, B. and Ellis, A., with Cheibub, J.A. (2005). *Electoral System Design: The New International IDEA Handbook.* Stockholm: IDEA

Sachs M. (2002). By Elections in 2001: A statistical Review. UMRABULO. Issue number 14 in aril ANC. www.anc.org.za/ancdocs/pubs/umrabulo/umrabulo14/elections.html

SADC HIV/AIDS Strategic Framework and Programme of Action (2003–7) Gaborone: SADC

SADC and International Cooperating Partners. (2006). Framework on Regional Support to HIV and AIDS in Southern Africa.

Schonteich, M. (2003a). "Impact and Mainstreaming of HIV and AIDS within Security Institutions," Pretoria: Institute for Security Studies.

Singh, K. (2003). Aid and Good Governance A Discussion Paper for The Reality of Aid Public Interest Research Group India

Strand, P., Matlosa, K., Strode, A. and Chirambo, K. (2005). *HIV/AIDS and Democratic Governance in South Africa: Illustrating the Impact on Electoral Processes.* Cape Town: IDASA.

United Nations. (2006). Scaling Up HIV Prevention, Treatment Care and Support.

UNAIDS (2003). *Epidemiological Update.* Geneva: UNAIDS.

UNAIDS/WHO global reports (2002–5)

UNDP/SADC Human Development Report (2000). Harare: SAPES Books.

UNDP (1997), "Reconceptualizing Governance", New York: UNDP, Discussion Paper 2.

UNDP (2002), "Deepening Democracy in a Fragmented World," Human Development Report 2002, New York: UNDP, also available on www.undp.org

Youde, J. (2001), *All the Voters Will be Dead: HIV/AIDS and Democratic Legitimacy and Stability in Africa.* University of Iowa.

2 Economic and social inequalities and HIV/AIDS in China

Implications for policy and governance

Dylan Sutherland

> Although many who study the dynamics of infectious disease will concede that, in some sense, disease emergence is a socially produced phenomenon, few have examined the contribution of specific social inequalities. Yet such inequalities have powerfully sculpted not only the distribution of infectious diseases but also the course of health outcomes among the afflicted.
>
> (Farmer 1999: 5)

This chapter considers whether better understanding the role of certain social inequalities, especially income inequalities, may help explain China's rapidly growing and evolving HIV/AIDS epidemic. Such understandings are important, as they may inform policy of the broader structural responses needed to combat an HIV/AIDS crisis and point to the type of governance mechanisms that are most suitable. There is little evidence, despite the scaling up of responses after the 2003 SARS epidemic, that Chinese policy makers have yet appreciated the magnitude and impact of these forces. Instead, a focus on information and education campaigns, following mainstream policy, appears to be the primary response. A range of studies, however, produced by researchers in a variety of disciplines using very different methods, now argues that a number of social and economic inequalities have a strong impact on population health [for some popular examples see Farmer (1999) and Wilkinson (2005)]. It is of particular importance that income inequality, given its rapid increase in China, has been found to have a strong association with population health in the both the developed and developing world (Pei and Rodriguez 2006: 1069; Wilkinson and Pickett 2006). As well as this and of great relevance to the current study at hand and the Chinese HIV/AIDS epidemic, recent empirical evidence also finds an extremely robust association between HIV/AIDS prevalence both income and gender inequalities (Drain *et al.* 2004; Talbott 2007; Nepal 2007; Crosby and Holtgrave 2003). Other studies, using different approaches (involving less quantitative analysis) make rather similar observations on the relationship between income and gender inequalities and HIV/AIDS epidemics (Barnett and Whiteside 2002; Kalipeni *et al.* 2004).

A strong association, then, has been established between income inequality and HIV/AIDS prevalence at the international level. This clearly raises important questions. Does such a relationship, for example, exist within countries at the sub-national level? Can we find such a relationship in China? If so, are the rapid and unprecedented increases in income inequality in China an important underlying factor explaining the emergence of the HIV/AIDS epidemic there? This chapter, building on other studies taking a so-called 'ecologic approach', attempts to answer some of these questions. More specifically, building on an established methodology, it tests empirically the relationships between income, gender inequality and a number of other important explanatory variables – including measures of gender inequality and a variety of other human development indicators (HDIs) – and HIV/AIDS prevalence. It asks what this may mean for policy as well as for governance responses.

The chapter is organised as follows. First, global and Asian trends towards increasing income inequality are reviewed, and the evidence on the strong links between income inequality and health noted. Second, working towards a method for investigating China's HIV/AIDS and inequality relationship, the evidence and methodology from ecologic studies on income inequalities and HIV/AIDS prevalence is explained. Much evidence, at the population level, now suggests a strong association between the two. A method for further exploring this relationship in China is explained and the possible nature of the causal mechanisms between HIV/AIDS and inequality are discussed. Third, a regional breakdown of HIV/AIDS infections is compared with a number of HDIs, with a view to better understanding the HIV/AIDS inequality relationship in China. Following this description, formal tests are carried out on 30 Chinese provinces. This is followed by a discussion of the results and their implications for policy and governance mechanisms.

Growing income inequalities and the health–inequality relationship

Before considering in more detail the evidence on the specific relationship between HIV/AIDS and income inequality, we note that the global trends in income distribution are worrisome. The World Bank's *World Development Report* 2006: *Equity and Development,* marked a milestone in the focus of World Bank research. For the first time, issues of equity were placed in the mainstream. A year later in 2007, the Asian Development Bank (ADB) produced a similar report, focusing on Asian inequality. Numerous other academic articles in the disciplines of economics and international development have also focused on this subject in recent times (Wade 2004). Their conclusions, on the whole, are quite negative concerning current trends: 'there is a growing sense that the impression of stable, unchanging income inequality may well be misleading' (World Bank 2006: 45). While it is difficult to obtain data, and measuring inequality across time and countries can also be problematic, data from 73 countries in the past two decades showed that 53 countries, encompassing 80 per cent of the world's population, saw increases in domestic inequality. Only four per cent have experienced decreases (UNDP 2005: 55).

While Asia's developing economies continue to grow at some of the fastest rates in the world, the concern today is that the poor are being bypassed by growth (ADB 2007: 87). As the World Bank notes:

> In general, the recent evidence in East Asia suggests that inequality has risen faster in the second round of high growth Asian economies – such as China and Vietnam – than had been observed in the first round – Hong Kong (China), Republic of Korea, Malaysia, Singapore, and Taiwan (China).
>
> (World Bank 2006: 45)

Indeed, relative inequality in many Asian countries between the early 1990s to and the early 2000s increased. Gini coefficients (a measure of inequality of income distribution ranging from 0, absolute equality, to 100, absolute inequality) for both incomes and expenditures, for example, increased in 15 out of 21 ADB member countries (ADB 2007: 87). Very large increases took place in Bangladesh, Cambodia, China, Lao PDR, Nepal and Sri Lanka. At an aggregate level in Asia, the share of income of the poorest 25 per cent of the population fell from 7.3 per cent in 1990 to 4.5 per cent in 2004. By contrast, in Sub-Saharan Africa the share of income of the bottom 25 per cent remained the same at 3.4 per cent (ADB 2007).

In China's case, the Gini coefficient has risen precipitously. In 1981, China was a relatively egalitarian society: the Gini coefficient was 28.8 according to the World Bank (World Bank 1997: 7). Its level of inequality was similar to that of Finland, the Netherlands, Poland and Romania. By 1996 China's income inequality had become roughly average by international standards. According to one study, it was 38.8 – 'lower than in most Latin American, African, and East Asian countries and similar to that in the United States, but higher than in most transition economies in Eastern Europe and many high-income countries in Western Europe' (World Bank 1997: 7). Even at this time, however, the increase in China's Gini coefficient was by far the largest of all countries for which comparable data were available: 'such a large change is unusual' (World Bank 1997: 3). There is general agreement China's income distribution 'has become much more unequal' (Naughton 2007: 209). By 2004, it had reached around 47, coming closer to the much higher figures typically associated with Latin America (ADB 2007: 87). As well as having the highest Gini coefficient in Asia, the ADB also found that spending by the wealthiest 20 per cent compared to the bottom quintile of the population in China increased faster than of any Asian country (ADB 2007). Worryingly, there is also some evidence that inequalities represented by extremes at the tails of the income distribution are particularly conducive to HIV/AIDS spread (UNAIDS 2006).The exact reasons for growing inequality remain controversial, and cannot be discussed at length here. China's rural–urban income gap, however, has recently been particularly large by international standards, and may be a major contributor. Urban incomes are rarely more than twice rural incomes, and in most countries rural incomes are around two-thirds or more of urban incomes. In China, however, rural incomes were only 40 per cent of urban incomes in 1995, down from a peak of 59 per cent in 1983, and this figure has decreased since (World Bank 1997: 15). By around 2005, urban incomes were around 3.2 times those of rural incomes. These figures, moreover, do not take into account differential increases in cost of living in rural and urban regions. Growing inequality is of direct relevance to these countries' overall population health and also, as will be shown, probably to the trajectory of their HIV/AIDS epidemics. Indeed, China's rural–urban inequalities are large by international standards. Only limited international comparative data on urban–rural income inequality exists. The International Labor Organization only publishes the ratio between per capita income from non-farm occupations and income from farming. Although this ratio is not entirely identical to urban–rural income inequality, it is quite close. In the 1990s, among eight countries whose ratio exceeded 2:1 were Botswana (3.02:1, 1995), Kenya (2.86:1, 1990) and Malawi (4.33:1, 1990), Zimbabwe (3.57:1) and South Africa (3.14:1) – all with serious generalized HIV/AIDS epidemics (CDRF and UNDP 2005: 27). There may be a particular relationship between HIV/AIDS and rural–urban income inequalities, though this is as yet unproven.

The government response to growing income inequality in China has taken place at a number of levels and with increasing urgency in recent years as social tensions have mounted. Measures to target around 600 impoverished areas, for example, were put in place, as were attempts to create a more comprehensive social security system. Programmes for developing the poorer western regions, including infrastructure development, were implemented. As well as this, taxes on farmers and fees levied on education and healthcare costs by local governments in rural areas have also been reduced. The top Chinese leadership also embraced a new 'scientific concept of development', a concept more akin to the idea of human development promoted by the UNDP (including aspects of health, education, gender issues, the environment and income). Efforts to curb corruption have been launched and monopolistic sectors of the economy have also been targeted for greater monitoring. Despite these various measures, however, income inequality has continued to increase, causing consternation to China's leaders.

One of the most interesting and remarkable insights of modern public health and social epidemiology is the discovery of the association between population health and income inequality. It has been observed that the international relationship between per capita income and life expectancy grows progressively weaker across countries as they get richer and 'disappears altogether among the wealthiest countries' (Wilkinson and Pickett, 2006: 1774). In wealthy nations, income inequalities become far better at explaining health outcomes than individual risk factors such as genetics and diet. It is argued in these countries that the social gradient in health within countries is primarily a gradient in relative income, or social status, rather than a reflection of absolute material living standards. Even in poorer countries, such as China, there is evidence that income inequality affects individual health, even after controlling for other individual factors (such as income, for example). Pei and Rodriguez (2006) test the relation between self-reported health and income inequality (using the Gini coefficient) with data from nine provinces in 1991, 1993 and 1997. Their results show an increased risk of about 10–15 per cent on average for fair or poor health for people living in provinces with greater income inequalities compared with provinces with modest income inequalities. It is of interest to note, furthermore, that the effect of income inequality on health intensified from 1991 to 1993 to 1997 as inequalities grew. It is now well established that income inequalities, which are growing especially quickly in many Asian countries, strongly affect health outcomes. The next section considers evidence on the relationship between a specific infectious disease (HIV/AIDS), income inequality and other population level social and economic indicators, with a view to developing methods which may help in better understanding the inequality/HIV/AIDS relationship in China.

Income and gender inequality and HIV/AIDS

Income distribution and changes in income distribution have been identified by a number of different researchers using different research methods as being of great importance in understanding HIV/AIDS epidemics [see, for example, Barnett and Whiteside (2002); Farmer (1999); as well as a range of 'ecologic' studies such as Talbott (2007), Drain *et al.* (2004) and Halperin and Bailey (1999)]. Indeed, a consideration of cross-sectional evidence on the correlation of adult HIV/AIDS prevalence and the Gini coefficient vividly illustrates this phenomenon. Figure 2.1 is a sample of 57 countries (including China and all other countries with similar or lower HDIs with available data). A statistically significant relationship exists between HIV/AIDS prevalence and income inequality in this sample, a finding that is repeated in numerous other studies (though, interestingly, it becomes weaker as higher HDI countries are included in the sample).

To further explore the relationship between HIV/AIDS and inequality, an understanding of recent research in this area is useful. Ecologic studies arguably provide some of the most important evidence for the relationship between income inequality and HIV/AIDS epidemics at the population level, which is the interest of this study. Indeed, the purpose of these studies, in large part, is to better understand the influence of societal characteristics on HIV transmission. By doing so, insights on population-level interventions may be found. Equally as importantly, recent studies also provide insights into approaches and methods that could be used to investigate the relationship between HIV/AIDS with inequality and other economic and sociocultural factors in China. This section, therefore, briefly reviews this useful

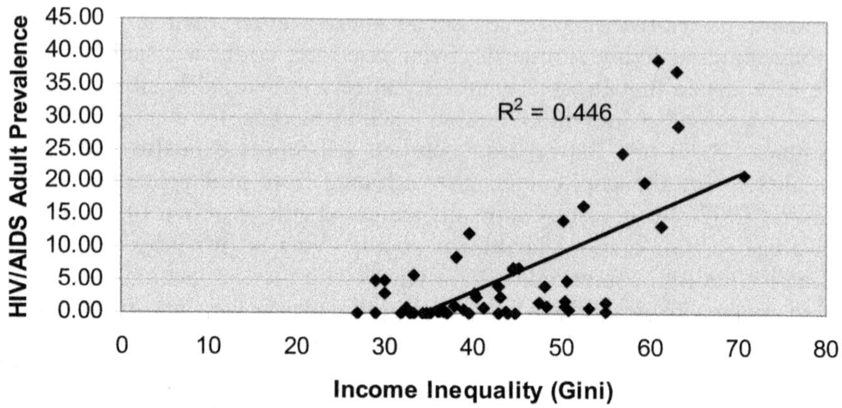

Figure 2.1 HIV prevalence and income distribution
Source: based on data reported in the UNDP Human Development Report (2005).

literature, before applying some of the methods to China's province-level data in the next section.

Ecologic studies

Ecologic studies provide statistical analyses of the interrelationships between HIV/AIDS and a variety of explanatory variables, often using large international data sets. Many of these studies, though not all, often begin by looking for statistical associations between a dependent variable (often some measure of HIV prevalence) and a range of possible explanatory variables. From this initial bivariate analysis, multivariate models are then specified. These studies, while having limitations, have at times proved quite powerful. Drain *et al.* (2004), for example, identified male circumcision as being associated with lower HIV prevalence using an ecologic study. Subsequent clinical trials in Uganda and Kenya confirmed that male circumcision does indeed appear to reduce the chances of HIV infection. Ecologic analyses are therefore useful, as they help identify the economic and social determinants of HIV/AIDS epidemics within population groups (as opposed to individuals). Evidence of specific associations and even causality between different variables, when confirmed by a number of studies, provides help in thinking about the economic and social determinants of HIV/AIDS epidemics. Indeed, such ecologic studies now consistently find that only a small number of variables are associated with adult HIV prevalence both at the national and even the subnational level; income and gender inequalities are among the two most important.

Table 2.1 summarises some of the findings of relevant studies. Over (1998), in an early study, looked at urban population groups, and examines the

Table 2.1 Summary of some ecologic studies on HIV/AIDS, including explanatory variables included and samples used.

Study	*Size of sample*	*Year of study*	*Country sample type*	*Main data source of sample (on HIV/ AIDS prevalence, for example)*	*Income inequality (significant – yes/no)*	*Gender inequality (significant – yes/no)*	*Types of some other explanatory variables also investigated (significant –yes/no)*
Drain *et al.* (2004)	122 countries	2000	Low HDI	UNAIDS, UNDP	Yes	Yes	Examine 81 different socioeconomic/development variables
Talbott (2007)	77 countries		Both low and high HDI samples	UNAIDS, UNDP	Yes (Gini)	Yes (significant)	Muslim faith, female/male illiteracy difference
Nepal (2007)	Developed and developing countries	2000	Both low and high HDI samples	UNAIDS, UNDP	Yes (Gini)	Yes (significant)	Governance (Yes)
Over (1998)	72 countries	1997	Developing countries	US Census Bureau	Yes (Gini)		13 variables
Holtgrave and Crosby (2003)	US states	1999	United States	Federal surveillance documents.	Yes (richest/ poorest deciles)	Not tested	Social capital, poverty
Moran and Jordaan (2007)	Russian regions	2002	Russia		No		Per capita wealth, population mobility (income inequality?), drug use, healthcare, age of epidemic
This study	30 Chinese provinces	2005	China – low and medium HDI provinces	UNAIDS, China Ministry of Health, China Development Research Foundation/UNDP	Yes (significant)	Yes (significant)	Education, rural/urban income gap, female illiteracy

Source: Drain *et al.* (2004); Nepal (2007); Holtgrave and Crosby (2003), Moran and Jordaan (2007).

influence of 13 variables for 72 countries. The age of the epidemic, GNP per capita and Gini index were most strongly correlated with HIV prevalence (after adjusting for other variables). This study also found a significant relationship with education differences between sexes. Drain *et al.* (2004), in widely cited research, undertake regression analyses for 122 developing countries using 81 different socioeconomic and developmental variables. Only several variables, however, of the variables that had enough data gathered to make meaningful comparisons, were significant in predicting HIV/AIDS levels in both linear and multiple regressions. These included: i) the Gini coefficient; ii) the percentage of a country's population that are of the Muslim faith; and iii) the percentage of a country's young adult (15–24 years old) women that are illiterate. Other variables that were found to be significantly correlated with HIV/AIDS prevalence were either measuring a result of high HIV prevalence such as life expectancy, or represented sexual behaviour variables for which limited data was available (Talbott 2007: 2). Drain *et al.* (2004) find no relationship with education inequalities between sexes.

Talbott (2007), using a different specification but building upon insights of earlier studies (by incorporating income and gender inequality and education), refutes some of the findings of Drain *et al.* (2004), and questions their method, in particular the weighting of countries by population. Talbott instead carries out cross-country linear and multiple regressions using newly gathered data from UNAIDS but this time with unweighted populations, also including the number of female commercial sex workers (hereafter CSW) as a percentage of the female adult population as an explanatory variable and using a different sample (including both developed and developing countries). Talbott argues the previous findings of Drain *et al.* (2004) should be treated with care, as:

> In effect, they make data from China 400 times more weighted in their analysis than that from small population Botswana, an error that leads to many false conclusions. There is no reason to think that China's reported data is any more accurate than Botswana's and in trying to uncover possible government and social action that could correlate with HIV it makes no sense to weight one country's experiences or attempts more highly than another. More populous countries do not necessarily conduct more or better testing of their CSW populations.
>
> (Talbott 2007: 2)

Talbott's work, it should be noted, even when incorporating CSW and using the unweighted sample, actually confirms some of the findings of earlier studies. In particular it finds that female illiteracy levels, gender illiteracy differences and income inequality within countries are significantly and positively correlated with HIV/AIDS prevalence. CSW, moreover, is robustly positively correlated with countrywide HIV/AIDS prevalence levels. When CSW is incorporated in the model, the finding, at least at the population level, that the Muslim faith variable/circumcision reduces HIV prevalence is rejected. It is argued, however, that the Muslim faith reduces HIV prevalence via its influence in reducing the size of the commercial sex industry.

Nepal (2007) undertakes further cross-country regression analysis, building on previous studies but looking at both adult HIV prevalence as well as the percentage of women among adults living with HIV/AIDS, thus specifically addressing the feminisation of HIV/AIDS. Nepal includes both developed and developing countries in the sample. The estimates on HIV/AIDS prevalence provided by UNAIDS are the 'best ever' (ibid.: 5). Nepal finds in preliminary analysis a significant correlation with wealth, economic equity, gender equity and good governance. Further multivariate linear regression analysis, when accounting for collinearity among explanatory variables, identified economic and gender equity in particular as the two most important factors linked with the HIV/AIDS epidemic. Thus gender equity, when measured using the gender related development index, emerged as a 'consistently significant' determinant of the overall epidemic and the female epidemic as well (ibid.: 1). It is therefore argued that good governance and wealth, while being important, are not key: instead economic and gender equity were found to be much more important factors in determining the overall level of feminisation of the HIV/AIDS pandemic: 'gender equality appears to be a consistently significant correlate of both the HIV/AIDS pandemic and its female face' (ibid.: 4). The main findings, moreover, agree with some past ecological analysis conducted among developing countries (Drain *et al.* 2004).

Two national-level ecologic studies, looking at the national determinants of HIV/AIDS epidemics, also provide some insights into the economic and social determinants of HIV/AIDS epidemics. Crosby and Holtgrave (2003), for example, investigate the relationship between social capital and HIV/AIDS and other sexually transmitted diseases (STDs) in the United States. They complement other work that has related social capital to a number of important public health variables. As poverty and income inequality are closely related to, and thought to be important factors explaining the observed strength of social capital and health outcomes, they also consider poverty and inequality. They obtained state-level data and examined the relationship with poverty, income inequality/social capital and four STDs (Crosby and Holtgrave 2003: 62). They find that social capital (as measured by 14 variables included in Putnam's public use data set) was the only significant predictor for gonorrhea and syphilis. The variance explained by this social capital measure for these two, moreover, was quite large (45 per cent and 34.9 per cent respectively). For AIDS case rates, however, both social capital and income inequality were significantly correlated. The greater the social capital, the lower the AIDS case rate; and the more income inequality, the higher the AIDS case rate (ibid.: 63). While there is debate as to the exact definition and nature of social capital, and its evolution in China is not greatly researched, it may be possible that our measure of Chinese income inequality, considered shortly, also captures changes in social capital. This is based on the observation that other studies have noted the close relationship between social capital and income inequality (Wilkinson 2005).

Finally, Moran and Jordaan (2007) look at Russia, and identify four main factors influencing HIV prevalence in Russian regions. These factors all consist of elements that represent the processes of economic and social development. They find that urbanisation, mobility, crime and income growth are important factors. They do not, unfortunately, explicitly test for inequality, which is strange given the strong associations found in previous studies. The strong statistical relationships that they uncover, however, still point towards the strong impact of social and economic development patterns on the trajectory of the epidemic. They argue that economic and social forces cannot be ignored in constructing policy.

Ecologic studies on HIV/AIDS prevalence are increasing in number. They point towards a number of explanatory variables that could be used to further investigate population-level HIV/AIDS prevalence. In particular, income and gender inequality emerge quite consistently as having a strong association and statistical significance in multivariate analysis of HIV/AIDS prevalence [covering different time periods and samples (as shown in Table 2.1)]. These studies, moreover, also suggest several possible methods that might be used for examining the relationship in China. Based on the insights and methods of these studies, this chapter explores in more detail the HIV/AIDS and income/gender inequality relationship in China at the sub-national level. Before this, however, it is worth further speculating as to why income and gender inequalities as measured at the population level may be important in causing China's HIV/AIDS epidemic.

Untangling causal mechanisms: why is income and gender inequality important?

First of all, it is important to note that inferring causality from ecologic studies remains problematic, owing to the inherent difficulties of such estimation procedures. Crosby and Holtgrave (2003), for example, note that their analysis does not allow them to infer definitive causal associations. Moran and Jordaan (2007) admit their variables are measured at a high level of aggregation and represent diverse processes within regions. Urbanisation, for example, is likely to represent the composite effect of many factors (ibid.: 8). Within the vast literature on the health–inequality relationship in developed countries, moreover, a key debate exists as to what exactly income inequality really reflects (Wilkinson and Pickett 2006). Thus, even though a relationship between certain variables may be established, the exact nature and mechanisms of causal processes may remain rather vague. It is not the specific purpose of this chapter to investigate in detail the causal mechanisms. Briefly, however, we mention some areas that research has highlighted and that would seem to be of importance in the Chinese case. We first consider income, then gender inequality.

First, it is clear that income inequality itself is closely associated with numerous other factors that may individually, or working together, predispose populations to high risk. Changes in income distribution, for example, may occur as a result of the overall development process. As Kuznets (1954) hypothesised, an inverted U-shape relationship may exist between inequality and income. Growing inequality occurs in early stages of growth because differences between rural and urban areas become more pronounced as industrialisation gets underway. It is only as the new urban migrant classes become assimilated to the working and middle classes and start to participate politically that income distributions again become more even. According to this interpretation, inequality is intimately related to the entire development process – industrialisation, urbanisation, large-scale migration, evolving state-society relations, governance, social and political change, etc.

Clearly, migration from rural to urban areas and the creation of a class of disenfranchised migrant workers predisposed to high-risk behaviour is integral to this development process and also central to understanding HIV/AIDS in China. Over 100 million migrants now exist, with limited access to healthcare, lower levels of education and income, habitual insecurities and psychosocial stresses. The feminisation of migration and labour markets, moreover, is an ongoing process (Gaetano and Jacka 2004; Zhang, Brauw and Rozelle 2004). In China, it is particularly noticeable that not only has a feminisation of migration taken place, but also that the average age of female migrants has fallen considerably (more and more women in their teens and early twenties are migrating).This has undoubtedly contributed to the boom in CSWs (as it did also in Thailand), something that few leaders in China have yet to publicly acknowledge. The sex industry itself is driven by extremely favourable demand-side (growing urban male middle classes) and supply-side conditions (growing gender inequalities in health and education, lack of poverty reduction in rural areas, weak legal systems and deeply corrupt local governments) (Pan Suiming 1999).

Income inequalities drive migration and, also, the sex industry – the economic and social bases of the latter are becoming increasingly well understood (Lin 1998). China, like Thailand, which itself also experienced similar precipitous increases in inequality, has a very large sex industry (with possibly over five million workers at any single time). This sector itself also experiences a large turnover as the young females in the sex sector, generally, see it only as a short-term occupation, a period of transition after which they can move on to better things. The future of the battle against HIV/AIDS in China, most probably, lies in combatting the activities of the commercial sex sector. This, in turn, is closely related to the particular pattern of economic development and coupled with growing gender inequalities (which themselves tend to be greater in poor regions with high levels of income inequality). Talbott (2007), in one of the few papers to accommodate the sex industry in estimates of HIV prevalence, shows just how important commercial sex work is to an understanding of HIV/AIDS epidemics.

Other studies have also pointed to the relationship between income inequality and poverty (UNAIDS 2006). Other things being equal, higher income inequality is likely to exacerbate poverty. For any given amount of growth, poverty reduction will be reduced in unequal societies: 'AIDS has been exacerbated by deepening poverty experienced by the majority of African countries over the past 20 years' (Craddock 2004: 5). And, it should be added, the growing levels of inequality in income accompanying these countries' development. Poverty may in turn be related to poor health, untreated STDs, lower levels of nutritional intake and in turn greater susceptibility (Stillwaggon 2006). This is particularly true in China, where poverty reduction has been dramatic but highly uneven and coupled with huge reductions in central public expenditure on health. From 1981 to 2001, the number of people living in poverty fell from 53 to eight per cent – a massive reduction (Ravallion and Chen 2004: 16). About half of the entire decline, however, took place in the first few years of the 1980s and poverty reduction stalled in the late 1980s and early 1990s, recovered in the mid 1990s but then stagnated again later in the decade. Some household survey studies find that, after initially rising, the absolute living standards of the poor declined considerably from 1995 to 1999. At this time they were again approaching income levels of 1987: 'as much as half of all households were not unambiguously better off in 1999 than in 1987: *the rising tide did not lift all boats*' (Benjamin, Brandt and Giles 2005: 771). This is most worrying. According to one UNAIDS publication, the relationship between poverty and inequality is 'powerful but nuanced' (UNAIDS 2006: 84):

> In the most affected countries (prevalence over 20 per cent – all in southern Africa), the richest 10 per cent of the population have revenues that are almost 70 times those of the poorest 10 per cent of the population. This compares with much lower disparities or ratios of between 20 and 27 in countries with lower prevalence. On average, one-third of the population in the most-affected countries with high income disparity lives on less than US$1 per day – a large proportion, given their relatively high gross domestic product.
>
> (UNAIDS 2006: 84)

In this analysis, the most affected countries are not necessarily the poorest but rather the ones with especially large gaps between the very poorest and richest. Southern Africa, with the world's highest HIV prevalence, includes the most economically developed countries in Sub-Saharan Africa. Generally, these countries have higher levels of education, gross domestic product, and access to water and sanitation than other parts of the continent. They also tend, however, to have greater economic inequality and, in particular, large gaps between the richest and poorest, with large numbers of people living in poverty. Within Asia, China now has one of the largest gaps between the richest and poorest deciles, which does not bode well for its HIV/AIDS epidemics (ADB 2007).

Others have argued that a skewed income distribution may have impacts via its affect on social capital and cohesion. Barnett and Whiteside, for example, argue that the existence of a risk environment reflects 'the breakdown of social order and cohesion' (Barnett and Whiteside 2002: 92). Closely related to social cohesion are issues of sexual mixing patterns. It has been noted, for example, that a relationship may exist between the degree of social order and sexual mixing patterns between groups. In periods of rapid economic change, where 'livelihoods are uncertain either because of growth or decline[,] people's livelihood strategies may facilitate faster change of sexual partners within and between diverse groups' (ibid.: 92). Social capital and cohesion may also have an impact via drug addiction. These ideas are supported by research for the United States (Crosby and Holtgrave 2003).

Gender inequalities, as well as those in income, are now also generally considered key to understanding HIV/AIDS. The interrelationship between development and gender is now a much researched area, as are the specific characteristics of these relations in transition economies (Beneria 2003). When it comes to HIV/AIDS, it is considered that various gender inequalities, such as in access to education, income, political rights, as well as cultural biases, put females at risk. They may be forced into dangerous relationships and, as importantly, into lifestyles that inherently pose greater dangers. This is particularly evident in China, where the massive commercial sex market has also been driven by the gender inequalities pervasive in Chinese society. Since economic reforms in the 1980s, there is much evidence to suggest that various forms of gender inequality have been on the rise (in income, education and health in particular) [see Berik, Dong and Summerfield (2007) for a good summary]. In the labour market, for example, considerable wage segmentation has emerged between males and females, as has access to capital and participation in ownership. Women are less likely to have pensions (in urban areas) and more likely to be laid off. Considerable wage discrimination also exists in rural township and village enterprises. Poverty has therefore also become feminized, with more and more of China's poor being females. Owing to discrimination in rural areas (less access to education, medical care and food, the adverse impacts of land reform on land ownership for females) women are, in the final analysis, prepared to migrate to urban areas for a lower wage than men, again increasing the financial motivation for alternative employment such as sex work. Indeed, it seems quite possible that the most immediate threat that gender inequalities pose in China are related to their role in driving the commercial sex industry. Lack of education, political empowerment to affect change, access to better employment and healthcare (which has also deteriorated as a result of market reforms) must also, however, play important parts. The reduced access to healthcare, in particular, has led to a dramatic resurgence in STDs (illustrated, for example, by the explosion in syphilis cases), which in turn greatly speed the spread of HIV.

There are numerous mechanisms through which inequalities in income and gender may drive the HIV/AIDS epidemic in China. Here we have considered a few. Among arguably the most important in China, however, are the impacts on population mobility, gender inequalities, health care and education provision. Closely related to all of these, moreover, is the emergence of a massive commercial sex market (facilitated by widespread corruption). As the epidemic matures and establishes itself more firmly in heterosexual networks, it is possible the relationship between income inequality and HIV/AIDS prevalence may even strengthen. Having reviewed some of the findings of the ecologic literature, and considered the possible relationship between income, gender inequality and HIV/AIDS, we now look to further test this question using a similar ecologic approach to those discussed earlier. In this case, however, we look to use data gathered from China's provinces.

HIV/AIDS and inequality in China: Testing an ecologic approach

We have established that strong statistical associations exist between economic and social inequalities, particularly those related to income and gender, and that there are also reasons for thinking these inequalities may themselves be causal in the HIV/AIDS epidemics. To test the relationship between HIV/AIDS prevalence and economic and social development variables, however, a number of candidates present themselves (see Table 2.1 for some examples of these). To recap, the Gini coefficient, the percentage of a country's young adult population that are Muslim, the percentage of country's young adult women that are illiterate, the difference between the young female and male illiteracy rates and the size of CSW are among just some of the variables that have been found to be significant predictors of HIV/AIDS prevalence at the population level (see Table 2.1). Talbott (2007), for example, finds that approximately 45 per cent of the variance in HIV could be explained in his model (ibid.: 4). Examination of the studies presented in Table 2.1, however, suggests that two variables appear to emerge most consistently as being strongly associated with HIV/AIDS prevalence: those related to income and gender inequality. While for the purposes of this study, CSW would also be an interesting variable to explore, such estimates do not exist. Similarly, the Muslim religion is likely to appear of marginal importance in explaining HIV/AIDS in China given the relatively small number of Muslims (Xinjiang, however, a Muslim region, also has among the highest prevalence).

This section explores and tests these variables for China, using a comparative as well as ecologic approach at the provincial level (i.e. sub-national). First, high-prevalence provinces (with greater than one per cent of China's total HIV/AIDS infections) are scrutinised for possible relationships between various HDIs (such as education and health) and HIV/AIDS prevalence. We create a high-prevalence sample allowing quick comparisons to be made (Table 2.2).

Second, the sample is tested and then expanded (to include 30 as opposed to 15 of China's provinces) and multivariate regression analysis is used to explore possible relationships for the full sample. The more parsimonious model of Nepal (2007) is used to test both the full and reduced sample.

Table 2.2 Human development and HIV/AIDS infections in China

Region	*a.*	*Total HDI*	*HDI Rank*	*Population*	*Urban per capita GDP*	*Rural per capita GDP*	*Urban/ rural*	*b.*	*Illiteracy rate*	*Male illiteracy (%)*	*Female illiteracy (%)*	*Illiterate females / males*	*c.*	*d.*	*e.*
China		0.75							10.9	6.1	15.9	2.6	98.7	55.4	28.6
Shanghai	1.1%	0.91	1	17.11	49946	22353	2.2	3.2	5.88	2.14	9.6	4.5	99.6	91.5	57.4
Beijing	1.8%	0.88	2	14.56	37031	14942	2.5	0.7	4.61	1.96	7.41	3.8	99.6	87.6	68.3
Tianjin		0.85	3	10.11	31437	13919	2.3	6.7	6.36	2.97	9.62	3.2	99.6	79.3	51.9
Guangdong	8.3%	0.81	6	79.54	24683	8084	3.1	0.7	7.55	3.06	12	3.9	99.4	47.8	25.9
High HDI Total	11.2%		Averages	121.32	35774.3	14824.5	2.5		6.1	2.5	9.7	3.9	99.6	76.6	50.9
Xinjiang	8.3%	0.76	14	19.34	18221	5350	3.4	6.1	6.94	5.32	8.62	1.6	96.2	49.8	18.2
Hubei	2.0%	0.76	15	60.02	14732	5164	2.9	5.6	11.83	5.77	17.99	3.1	99.2	58.5	37.9
Shanxi	1.0%	0.75	16	33.14	13214	4337	3.0	7.1	5.79	3.34	8.32	2.5	99.3	71.4	26.3
Hunan	1.9%	0.75	17	66.63	14279	4713	3.0	3.6	8.47	4.51	12.67	2.8	98.2	60.6	32.2
Chongqing	1.3%	0.75	18	31.3	14024	3837	3.7	4.0	8.4	4.42	12.4	2.8	95.4	59.3	39.5
Total medium HDI Total	14.5%		Averages	210.43	14894.0	4680.2	3.2		8.3	4.7	12.0	2.6	97.7	59.9	30.8
Henan	21.4%	0.74	19	96.67	15774	5092	3.1	8.3	9.21	5.13	13.37	2.6	99.2	43.2	14.1
Guangxi	12.2%	0.73	22	48.57	12581	3385	3.7	3.0	8.85	4.28	13.72	3.2	98.1	41.8	14.6
Sichuan	4.5%	0.73	24	87	12859	4072	3.2	4.7	11.73	7.06	16.42	2.3	95.8	55	32.1
Anhui	2.7%	0.73	25	64.1	12792	4015	3.2	2.9	13.67	7.76	19.72	2.5	99.3	59	21.3
Yunnan	26.0%	0.66	29	43.76	14012	3111	4.5	3.7	21.5	13.84	29.81	2.2	98	35.8	13.3
Guizhou	2.1%	0.64	30	38.7	8573	2042	4.2	5.0	19.68	11.97	27.72	2.3	97	39.5	15.3
Total low HDI	67.3%		Averages	378.8	12765.2	3619.5	3.6		15.1	9.0	21.5	2.5	97.9	45.7	18.5

Source: China Human Development Report 2005.

Notes: a. share of total cumulative HIV infections in China end of 2005; b. poverty (% beneath poverty line); c. primary school enrolments; d. high school enrolments; e. university and college.

Following Drain *et al.* (2004) and Crosby and Holtgrave (2003), a variety of different bivariate associations between HIV/AIDS prevalence and social and economic development indicators are then also examined. A number of alternative models are also specified and tested to examine the robustness of income inequality.

Data and sources

Province-level data on HIV/AIDS prevalence has been estimated by China's Ministry of Health (based on data collected from sentinel surveillance sites by local and central disease control centres), and is reported by UNAIDS China as well as the Ministry of Health. In recent years, as more surveillance sites representing lower risk populations have been included, downward revisions have been made. This analysis uses the more recent estimates, as reported by Lu *et al.* (2006). These estimates are given in terms of total infections estimated within certain bounds – they are therefore not specific. From these bounds, mid-points are taken and province-wide prevalence is estimated using population figures from the China Statistical Yearbook. The results are also cross-checked against earlier estimates of adult prevalence to check for consistency of results. Earlier estimates are expressed in prevalence per 10,000 people (see Qian, Vermund and Wang 2005).

All other human, economic and social development variables are taken from the China Human Development Report, 2005 (CDRF and UNDP 2005). As no Gini coefficients are available at the province level, income inequality is calculated using urban/rural income. Income inequality and distribution can, of course, be captured in numerous ways. Although the Gini coefficient is a common method of estimating inequality, this single aggregate figure can capture a wide variety of different income distributions. Two identical Gini coefficients, for example, may hide very different income distributions. Using the rural–urban income gap, however, may capture one particularly important element of Chinese inequality, as it has been suggested that rural–urban differences are central to understanding Chinese inequality (World Bank 1997). As also noted earlier, large rural-urban income gaps have been found in some of the highest-prevalence countries of Africa. On the other hand, some recent studies also show intraregional inequalities are of more importance to Chinese inequality than previously recognized (Benjamin, Brandt and Giles 2005). Thus using rural–urban differences may not fully capture the nature of income inequality in China, and intra-urban and intra-rural inequality may also be important. Measurements of female illiteracy and the male/female illiteracy differences are also constructed from the China Human Development Report. Poverty rates, various measures of educational attainment (university, high school and primary enrolment), the extent of industrialisation, unemployment, rural and urban human development indexes, per capita GDP and medical care are some other variables that are also investigated.

Data description and analysis

Table 2.2 provides summary details of some HDIs for provinces that are recorded as having over one per cent of the national total of HIV infections as reported by UNAIDS China for the end of 2005. The table provides information on 15 of the most affected provinces in China (our full sample contains 30 observations). It is worth briefly examining the regional HIV/AIDS situation to gain an overview and insights into the possible relationships between HIV/AIDS prevalence and human and social development indicators. The provinces are also broken down according to their HDI score (a composite measure, which equally weights income, health and education measures to provide an index of human development – a not uncontroversial measurement, but suitable enough for our current purposes of categorising provinces).

First, it is evident that the regions with lower levels of human development, even when accounting for their larger populations, generally have relatively more infections than other regions. Thus, Henan, Jiangxi, Guangxi, Sichuan, Anhui, Yunnan and Guizhou, which for the purposes of this table are recorded as low-HDI provinces (beneath 0.75) had 67 per cent of all recorded HIV infections in China by the end of 2005. Yunnan, Henan and Guangxi had the most infections in these provinces. In the provinces with a medium HDI score (for the purpose of this exercise with indicators ranging from 0.75 to 0.8, including Xinjiang, Hubei, Shanxi, Hunan and Chongqing) the cumulative number of infections reached 14.5 per cent of China's total. For the provinces with higher HDI scores (Shanghai, Beijing, Tianjin and Guangdong) the share of the national total of HIV infections stood at 11.2 per cent.

Second, there are wide disparities within provinces between rural and urban areas and these disparities vary between high- and low-HDI regions. In the low -HDI regions, for example, the average urban per capita income was ¥12,765 but only ¥3,619 in rural areas (3.6 times the rural level). In the medium human development regions urban per capita incomes were slightly higher (¥14,894) as were rural (¥4,680). The multiple between rural and urban was now close to the national average (at 3.2 times). In the regions with high HDI scores, incomes were higher (urban per capita incomes ¥35,774; rural ¥14,824) and the relative income difference between rural and urban areas also less (urban incomes were 2.5 those of rural). These figures show that areas with low HDI scores also have a greater difference between urban and rural areas.

Third, in terms of illiteracy, the low human development regions fared particularly badly. The average for the region saw 20 per cent illiteracy among females and nine per cent for males. The female illiteracy rate falls to 12 per cent in medium HDI regions and almost 10 per cent in developed regions. The male illiteracy rate falls from nine to 4.7 to 2.5 per cent as we move from low to high HDI regions. Interestingly, however, the ratio of male to female illiterates deteriorates as we make this move. Female illiteracy, other studies suggest, is of great significance for the understanding of HIV epidemics. The low levels of literacy more generally reflect gender discrimination and the lack of empowerment females may experience in these regions.

A comparison of China's regional HIV prevalence and HDIs reveals some insights into the inequality/HIV relationship. It would appear, among other things, that regions with greater income inequality and lower female literacy have higher rates of infection. Does this apparent relationship hold when undertaking a more formal statistical analysis?

Multivariate regression analysis

Following Nepal (2007), we first look to estimate a simple model that includes only our measure of income inequality and female education as measured by the female illiteracy rate. This model has the advantage of parsimony, which is important given our relatively small sample. It also has strong theoretical backing and empirical support. It has the disadvantage, however, of a possible relationship among the explanatory variables (i.e. there is a relationship between gender and income inequality variables, which could interfere with our results). We can, however, take this relationship into account by testing for this (see the later test descriptions). First, therefore, we make HIV prevalence our dependent variable and use the rural–urban gap and female illiteracy rate as explanatory variables (using the sample of provinces with more advanced epidemics). The results are shown in Table 2.3.

There are good reasons for restricting our sample to certain provinces, given the strong association between the age of the epidemic and prevalence that has been found elsewhere (Over 1998). It may be more sensible, for example, to only consider provinces in which epidemics are older and more established, given that the HIV/AIDS epidemics are still very much in their infancy in many Chinese provinces. Attempting to ascertain the impact of economic and social determinants in these provinces may be of less value. On the other hand, regions in which the epidemic is more established may better reflect the influence of social and economic factors. In this smaller sample, the coefficient on income inequality is significant at the five per cent level and that on female illiteracy at the 10 per cent level. The overall fit of our model appears to be quite good [as measured by the adjusted R^2, which is quite high (0.43)]. More formal testing procedures also confirm this (the F-test shows it

Table 2.3 HIV/AIDS prevalence by province on income inequality, female illiteracy, full and restricted samples

	Restricted sample	*Full sample*
Rural/Urban Gap	1.23**	8.75*
Female Illiteracy	0.42*	-0.29
Adjusted R squared	0.43	0.17

*Significant at 0.05 level, ** at 0.01 level.

to be significant at the one per cent level – this tests whether the overall model is a good fit, as opposed to testing individual explanatory variables which are shown in the table). Both the signs on the coefficient are as expected.[1] These results are of interest as they appear to quite closely correspond to the results of the previous ecologic studies already mentioned.

After testing this first sample, we go on to expand the sample to include all 30 provinces (primarily to increase the number of observations, which may provide more reliable statistical results). With this new sample, the coefficient of female illiteracy now becomes insignificant and has a coefficient contrary to that found in previous studies. Correlation, however, between the rural–urban income difference and female illiteracy (with an adjusted R^2 of 0.29 and significance at the one per cent level) is still quite high. The rural–urban gap, as noted, is highly related to female illiteracy – the greater the disparity between rural and urban regions, the higher the female illiteracy rate. This may, as discussed earlier, lead to estimation problems (by inflating the variances of our estimators, making them unreliable and known technically as multicollinearity). Although the estimation with the full sample is in fact statistically significant ($F = 3.97$) and income inequality is again significant at the five per cent level the overall fit is by no means as close as the smaller high-prevalence sample or the international cross-section presented earlier (which has an R^2 approaching 0.5, as shown in Figure 2.1).

Finally, following the procedures of previous ecologic studies [for example, Drain *et al.* (2004)], we test the robustness of the income and gender inequality variable to a number of different specifications, drawing from over 15 other explanatory variables using our full and restricted samples, as well as using alternative estimations of HIV/AIDS prevalence by province (based around UNAIDS/MOH data). While we do not report all the findings here, we note that our income inequality explanatory variable holds up strongly and is particularly robust to the inclusion of new variables.

Despite these interesting results, a salutary note of caution on the limitations of ecologic-type studies must be added. Attempting to infer causality from such studies, in particular, owing to the difficulties of such estimations (involving at times statistical issues briefly touched upon, such as multicollinearity, specification of the wrong model which may create biases, etc.), is not straightforward. Moreover, such analyses also look at population groups as a whole. They therefore do not inform us specifically about individual risk factors or causal associations – this is a most important point to keep in mind. HIV prevalence in a population group also reflects the cumulative effects of risky behaviours and exposure to the virus over a number of years. Care is therefore required in making inferences based on static cross-sections about epidemic dynamics. There are, moreover, also obvious issues in use of data for some of the variables used in these studies. While some data may be inaccurate, it is also true that measures of several key potential influences on the HIV/AIDS epidemic, including drug use and sexual networks, are far from complete or missing entirely. This limits what can and cannot be tested for. Our sample size, moreover, is limited to 30 provinces in China, which makes it rather a small sample. Smaller units of analysis warrant further investigation, not only to increase sample size, but also to investigate whether income inequalities within smaller units have similar impacts. Studies on health in the developed world find the health–inequality relationship starts to break down when smaller units are used.

These exploratory estimations and results, nonetheless, do suggest that income inequality is a strong predictor of HIV/AIDS prevalence not only across countries (in international samples) but also within China. There is also evidence that gender inequality may also play its part in China's HIV/AIDS epidemic. This should not be entirely surprising given similar findings found in other ecologic studies for other regions of the world.

Discussion and conclusions

To date, owing to the caution with which civil society and non-governmental organisations have been allowed to freely participate, responses to the HIV/AIDS epidemic in China have really been led by the government at different levels. After the SARS outbreak in 2003, these responses grew considerably. Greater resources were committed to the response and high-level political involvement was also brought to the campaigns. Many of these responses, however, have so far focussed on conventional strategies based around information and education, responses routed in biomedical approaches to the understanding of HIV/AIDS epidemics. This approach is most evident in the annual China updates published by the Chinese Ministry of Health and the UN Theme Group. Very little reference, if any at all, is made to social determinants, though there is considerable coverage of individual behaviour patterns (condom usage, frequency of visits to sex workers, etc.). To date then, less attention has been paid to the social and economic dynamics of the HIV/AIDS epidemic in China. If we are to concede, however, along with Farmer's (1999) observation quoted at the beginning of this chapter, that disease emergence is a socially produced phenomenon, this raises the question of what the contributions are of specific social inequalities? This chapter tries to make a start in better understanding this highly complex question.

Of arguably greatest importance, and following the highly robust relationship observed across countries, we find that a significant relationship between income inequality and HIV/AIDS prevalence can be found in China. We have not dwelt at length here upon the question of why our measure of income inequality exhibits this strong association, and clearly more needs to be done to unearth the exact mechanisms at work. Despite this omission, however, we can confidently conclude that the levels of inequality in China, which are typically 'strikingly stable over time within a given country', have grown greatly and at high speed (World Bank 1997: 8). They are likely, moreover, to continue to grow. Despite the government's best efforts, urban areas continue to forge ahead. There is also evidence to suggest that certain gender inequalities may also have increased. If the findings in this chapter are correct, and a relationship between income and gender inequality and HIV/AIDS exists, this will have implications for China's HIV/AIDS epidemics and also the types of governance responses required.

To date, NGOs and civil society movements have been allowed rather limited space to work. New and recent initiatives, however, have focused on facilitating greater contributions from NGOs. The findings of this research, however, suggest that responses to HIV/AIDS must reach beyond the domains of what may conventionally be regarded (at least in China, in any case) as HIV/AIDS-related interventions. Greater political freedoms with regard to addressing the wider sphere of social injustices, particularly as related to inequalities in the distribution of wealth, but also areas such as health and education (with due attention also to gender issues), will most likely also be necessary. Addressing these broader inequalities may be as important, if not even more important in the longer term, than the cognitive-type interventions already underway in the response to tackling HIV/AIDS. In terms of governance responses, therefore, this research suggests that, without the broader political freedoms needed to address many of the social inequalities emerging in China today, it may be difficult to address the key structural features responsible for the Chinese HIV/AIDS epidemic. To date, the Chinese government has had limited success in addressing the problem of growing income inequality and corruption. Wider political participation, involving greater openness, may be one of the few ways to address such deeply rooted problems.

While income inequality has been found to be important, other studies find female illiteracy and gender inequality, in particular, to have a strong association with HIV prevalence (Nepal 2007; Talbott 2007). In one of our samples, we also find a statistically significant relationship between gender inequality and HIV/AIDS prevalence. This suggests gender inequality may also be a very important factor in further explaining the Chinese epidemic. It is also quite evident that the number and share of female infections is increasing rapidly. The large commercial sex industry, so central to HIV/AIDS epidemics in other Asian countries, is also of central importance to understanding the future dynamics of China's HIV/AIDS epidemic. While some empirical work finds little cross-country evidence to relate CSW to gender inequality (Talbott 2007), the most detailed investigations of commercial sex in Southeast Asia show its development to be intimately related to overall income and gender inequalities (Lin 1998). Better understanding of the gender dimension of China's HIV/AIDS epidemic, and in particular how it interacts with the commercial sex sector, is still required. It is clear, therefore, that the female population still needs far greater political representation. Again, many aspects of gender inequality have worsened during the reform era; this is most noticeable, for example, in the manifestation of large inequalities in income, wealth and education between males and females. Government responses, in the form of legislation, have had little impact on such inequalities. Again, greater empowerment and voice will probably be required if these issues are to be properly addressed.

Finally, it is worth stressing that some studies find a limited association between per capita income levels and HIV/AIDS prevalence (Nepal 2007; Talbott 2007). While not reported in our results, we also find no strong association between per capita income and prevalence in the Chinese provinces sampled here. This finding is important for two reasons. First, all regions of China, both *wealthy* and *poor*, given similar levels of inequality and other risk factors, may be equally vulnerable to HIV/AIDS. Second, *economic growth per se*, which has been seen by policy leaders as a panacea for so many of China's ills, may not provide any solution to the rapidly expanding HIV/AIDS epidemic. Indeed, it is quite possible that growth, when unevenly balanced as it has been, provides the perfect economic and social environment for a disease such as HIV/AIDS to spread and thrive. Louis Pasteur, a 19th century founder of modern medicine remarked that 'the microbe is nothing; the terrain, everything'. It is becoming clear that the economic and social terrain of a rapidly developing China may be very conducive to the spread of HIV/AIDS. Policy-making, as well as focusing on interventions at the level of the individual, must be aware of the strong undercurrents against which such policies must fight. The current top-down approach, in which individuals are exhorted to change their risky behaviours, should be complemented with a greater appreciation of the broader structural parameters in which individuals function.

Notes

1 The variance inflation factor checks for multicollinearity and is also low in this case. The tests for model specification are also favourable.

Bibliography

ADB (Asian Development Bank) (2007). *Key Indicators 2007*, Philippines: ADB Manila.

Barnett, T. and Whiteside, A. (2002). *AIDS in the Twenty First Century*. New York: Palgrave Macmillan.

Beneria, L. (2003). *Gender, Development, and Globalization: Economics as if All People Mattered*. New York and London: Routledge.

Benjamin, D., Brandt, L. and Giles, J. (2005). 'The Evolution of Income Inequality in Rural China', *Economic Development and Cultural Change*, 53 (4):769.

Berik, G., Dong, X.Y. and Summerfield, G. (2007). 'China's Transition and Feminist Economics. *Feminist Economics*, 13(3–4): 1–33.

CDRF (China Development Research Foundation) and UNDP (2005). *China Human Development Report*. Available online http://www.undp.org.cn/downloads/nhdr2005/NHDR2005_complete.pdf (accessed 1st November 2007).

Craddock, S. (2004). 'Beyond Epidemiology: Locating AIDS in Africa' Kalipeni, E., Craddock, S., Oppong, R.J., Ghosh, J. *HIV/AIDS in Africa: Beyond Epidemiology. Oxford: Blackwell*

Crosby, R.A. and Holtgrave, D. R. (2003). 'HIV/AIDS and Inequality: what do we know?' *Sexually Transmitted Infections*, 79: 62–64.

Drain P.K, Smith J.S., Hughes J.P., Halperin D.T., Holmes K.K. (2004). 'Correlates of National HIV Seroprevalence. An Ecologic Analysis of 122 Developing Countries', *Journal of Acquired Immune Deficiency Syndrome,* 35: 4.

Farmer, P. (1999). *Infections and Inequalities: The Modern Plagues*, Berkeley and Los Angeles, CA: University of California Press.

Gaetano, A.M. and Jacka, T. (2004). *On the Move: Women in Rural-to-Urban Migration in Contemporary China*, New York: Columbia University Press.

Halperin D.T., Bailey R.C. (1999). 'Male circumcision and HIV infection: 10 years and counting', *Lancet* 354: 1813–15.

Kalipeni, E., Craddock, S., Oppong, R.J. and Ghosh, J. (2004). *HIV/AIDS in Africa: Beyond Epidemiology*, Oxford: Blackwell Publishing.

Kuznets, S. (1954). 'Economic Growth and Income Inequality', *American Economic Review*, 45: 1–28.

Lin, L.L. (1998). *The Sex Sector: The Economic and Social Bases of Prostitution in Southeast Asia*, Geneva: International Labour Office.

Lu, F.N., Wang, Z. Wu, X., Sun, Rehnstrom, J., Poundstone, K.,Yu, W. and Pisani, E. (2006). 'Estimating the number of people at risk for and living with HIV in China in 2005: methods and results', *Sexually Transmitted. Infections* 82: 87–91.

Moran, D. and Jordaan, J.A. (2007). 'HIV/AIDS in Russia: determinants of regional prevalence', *International Journal of Health Geographics*, 6 (22): 1–9.

Naughton, B. (2007). *The Chinese Economy: Transitions and Growth*, Cambridge, MA: The MIT Press.

Nepal, B. (2007). 'Prosperity, Equity, Good Governance and Health: Focus on HIV/AIDS Pandemic and Its Feminisation', *World Health Population*, October: 1–8.

Over, M. (1998). '*The effect of Societal Variables on Urban Rates of HIV Infections in Developing Countries*'. In M. Ainsworth *et al.*, (ed.), *Confronting AIDS: Evidence from the Developing World.* Brussels: European Commission.

Pan Suiming (1999). *Three Red Light Districts in China*. Beijing: Qunyan Publishing House.

Talbott, J.R. (2007). 'Size Matters: The Number of Prostitutes and the Global HIV/AIDS Pandemic', *PLoS ONE* 2(6): e543.

Pei, X. and Rodriguez, E. (2006). 'Provincial income inequality and self-reported health status in China during 1991–97', *Journal of Epidemiology and Community Health*, 60: 1065–69.

Qian, Z.H., Vermund, S.H., and Wang, N. (2005). 'Risk of HIV/AIDS in China: subpopulations of special importance', *Sexually Transmitted Infections,* 2005 (81): 442–7.

Ravallion, R. and Chen, S. (2004). 'Learning from China's success', *Finance and Development*, December 2004.

Stillwaggon, E. (2006). *AIDS and the Ecology of Poverty*, New York: Oxford University Press.

UNAIDS (2006). *AIDS Epidemic Update.* Geneva.

UNDP (2005). *Human Development Report*. United Nations, Geneva.

Vandepitte, J., Lyerla, R., Dallabetta, G., Crabbe F., Alary M. and Buve, A. (2006). Estimates of the number of female sex workers in different regions of the world. *Sexually Transmitted Infections*, 82 (Suppl III): iii18–iii25.

Wade, R.H. (2004). 'Is Globalization Reducing Poverty and Inequality?' *World Development*, 32 (4): 567–89.

Wilkinson, R. (2005). *The Impact of Inequality: How to make sick societies healthier*, Oxford: Routledge.

Wilkinson, R.G. and Pickett, K. (2006). Income inequality and population health: A review and explanation of the evidence. *Social Science and Medicine* 62: 1768–84.

World Bank (1997). *Sharing Rising Incomes*, Washington DC.

—— (2006). *World Development Report: Equity and Development*. New York: Oxford University Press.

World Health Organisation (2003). *Social determinants of health: the solid facts*. 2nd Edition. Geneva.

Zhang, L., De Brauw, A. and Rozelle, S. (2004). 'China's rural labor market development and its gender implications', *China Economic Review*, 15: 230–47.

Part II

Non-state actors, popular participation and mechanisms of accountable governance

3 Accountability and the right of everyone to the enjoyment of the highest attainable standard of physical and mental health

Helen Potts

Accountability is a distinctive, complex and central feature of human rights. In the context of human rights, accountability refers to the requirement of the state to fully comply with its obligations under the international and regional human rights treaties to which it is a party. Concrete cases of individuals and groups seeking government accountability show that the real challenge is to convert this legal commitment into specific measures of implementation. Despite the critical importance of accountability, little work has been done to explore its meaning and content in the context of the right of everyone to the enjoyment of the highest attainable standard of physical and mental health (the right to health or the right to the highest attainable standard of health). As a result, the notion of accountability is often seriously misunderstood. This chapter begins to explore this area and, while there remains much work to be done on the topic, this modest contribution will provide information on how to make accountability count in the right to health, and hence in HIV/AIDS governance.[1]

The chapter focuses on the relationship between the state (government and its agents) and rights holders. There are numerous and diverse organisations and arrangements that are involved in the right to health. This has occurred largely as a result of the trend in all regions of the world towards a reduction in the role of the state in delivery of health services. These numerous and diverse arrangements include bilateral and multilateral agreements, non-government organisations (NGOs), private national and international corporations, international financial institutions, individuals, families and communities. While the presence of these diverse arrangements makes addressing of violations of the right to health by the state complicated, the state remains ultimately accountable for guaranteeing the realisation of the right to health, as a matter of international human rights law. It is therefore more urgent than ever to address the complex issue of accountability of government for implementation of the right to health.

The chapter, divided into four sections, is an introduction to accountability in the context of the right to health. The first identifies the sources of the right to health at the national, regional and international levels. The second provides a brief review of the content of the right to health. The third addresses the component parts of accountability in the context of the right to health. Accountability in this context is intended to provide rights holders with an opportunity to understand how government has discharged its obligations, and also to provide an opportunity for government to explain its conduct. This process necessarily requires participation, monitoring and mechanisms to allow the explanation and understanding to take place. The fourth and last section therefore also describes these three components, as well as providing examples of the various accountability mechanisms that should be available at the national, regional and international levels. In addition, rights holders are entitled to remedies when there has been a failure on the part of government to fulfil its obligations pursuant to the right to health. Examples of the types of remedies that should be available to rights holders are also provided. The chapter concludes by suggesting which of the universal factors are required for accountability in the context of the right to health.

Sources of the right to health

The right to health can be found in laws at three different levels: international, regional, and national.

International

There are many international human rights treaties that recognize the right to health. Though first formulated in the World Health Organisation (WHO) Constitution (1946), the central formulation of the right to health is contained in Article 12 of the International Covenant on Economic, Social and Cultural Rights (ICESCR or the Covenant) (see below).

The right is also contained in international treaties that have been created to protect the human rights of particular groups, including the International Convention on the Elimination of All Forms of Racial Discrimination, Article 5(e)(iv); the International Convention on the Elimination of All Forms of Discrimination Against Women, Articles 11(1)(f), 12 and 14(2) b; and the Convention on the Rights of the Child (the Children's Convention), Articles 3 (3), 17, 23, 25, 28 and 32. These treaties highlight the preoccupation that human rights treaties have with people who are vulnerable to discrimination and marginalisation and may require special attention.

ICESCR, Article 12

1. The States Parties to the present Covenant recognize the right of everyone to the enjoyment of the highest attainable standard of health.
2. The steps to be taken by the State Parties to the present Covenant to achieve the full realization of this right shall include those necessary for:

(a) The provision for the reduction of the stillbirth-rate and of infant mortality and for the healthy development of the child;
(b) The improvement of all aspects of environmental and industrial hygiene;
(c) The prevention, treatment and control of epidemic, endemic, occupational and other diseases;
(d) The creation of conditions which would assure to all medical service and medical attention in the event of sickness.

Regional

In addition to international standards, the right to health is recognised in regional human rights treaties, including the African [Banjul] Charter on Human and Peoples' Rights, (Article 16); the African Charter on the rights and Welfare of the Child, (Article 14); the European Social Charter (Revised), (Article 11); and the Additional Protocol to the American Convention on Human Rights in the Area of Economic, Social and Cultural Rights (Protocol of San Salvador), (Article 10).

Other regional instruments, which do not explicitly recognize the right to health but which offer indirect protections through other health-related rights, include the American Declaration on the Rights and Duties of Man; the American Convention on Human Rights; the Inter-American Convention on the Prevention, Punishment and Eradication of Violence against Women; and the European Convention for the Protection of Human Rights and Fundamental Freedoms and its protocols.

National

The right to health is recognised in numerous national constitutions (Kinney and Clark 2004). When the right to health is enshrined in the constitution or in domestic laws, it creates an opportunity for an individual or group to pursue a complaint and seek a legally binding decision in the Courts if the right to health or another relevant right (e.g. the right to freedom from discrimination) has been violated. The right to health has also been indirectly protected in domestic courts through incorporation of the right into another human right. For example, the Supreme Court of India has, in several cases, found that social rights such as the right to health are an integral part of the fundamental rights guaranteed by the Constitution. See, for example, the case of *Paschim Banga Khet Mazdoor Samity and Ors v State of West Bengal* (1994).

Content of right to health

In recent years, an analytical framework has been developed with a view to making it easier to understand and apply to health-related policies.[2] The framework identifies 10 key elements of the right to health which have general application to all aspects of the right to health, including the underlying determinants of health.

i. National and international human rights laws, norms and standards

The laws and standards relevant to the particular policy must be identified. These will include both specific right to health provisions as well as general provisions. In addition, international and regional instruments that relate to specific groups and contexts must also be identified.

Progressive realisation

The right to health is subject to progressive realisation and resource constraints (ICESCR, 1976, article 2). Put simply, all countries are expected to be doing better in two years' time than they are today. Many countries do not currently have the capacity or the resources necessary to implement fully the right to health for all people. Nonetheless, governments must take deliberate and concrete steps toward the full realisation of the right to health for all. The corollary to the obligation to progressively realise the right to health is that 'there is a strong presumption that retrogressive measures taken in relation to the right to health are not permissible' (General Comment, No. 14, 2000, para.32). In order to measure progress (or the lack of it) over time, indicators and benchmarks must be identified (General Comment No. 14, 2000, paras. 57–58). While it is the government that has the obligation to develop indicators and benchmarks, indicators which measure progressive realisation can also be developed by civil society.[3]

Minimum core

In addition to the obligation to progressively realise the right to health, some core obligations are imposed with immediate effect. These core obligations require, at the very least, minimum essential levels of primary healthcare, food, housing, sanitation, essential drugs and the adoption and implementation of a national health strategy (General Comment No. 3 1990, para. 10; General Comment No. 14, 2000, para. 43). Even in the presence of limited resources, therefore, the government is required to give first priority to the most basic health needs of the population and to pay particular attention to protecting the most vulnerable sections of the population.

Freedoms and entitlements

The right to health encompasses both freedoms and entitlement. The freedoms include, for example, the right to make decisions about one's health, including sexual and reproductive freedom or non-consensual medical treatment and experimentation. The entitlements include, for example, the right to emergency medical services, and to the underlying determinants of health, such as adequate sanitation, safe water, adequate food and shelter, safe and healthy working conditions, and a healthy environment (General Comment No. 14, 2000, para. 8).

ii. Availability, accessibility, acceptability and quality

All health facilities, goods and services should comply with each of the four interrelated and essential elements of availability, accessibility, acceptability and quality (AAAQ, General Comment No. 14, para. 12).[4] Availability is concerned with the physical presence of health facilities, which must be available in sufficient quantities within the country. For example, availability is concerned with whether there is a sufficient number of health workers and health facilities in rural areas; whether there is a national public health plan; whether there is a health complaints commissioner or similar; and whether sexual and reproductive health services are provided. In regards to accessibility, health facilities must also be physically and economically accessible to everyone without discrimination, especially the most vulnerable or marginalized people. For example, while a health centre may be available at the local level, people in wheelchairs may not be able to access the centre because of the lack of wheelchair ramps, or the health workers may not speak the same language as the people attending the health centre. If the centre provides no physical access for people with a disability or no one at the facility speaks the local language then the facility is not accessible, even though it is available. If the facility charges user fees and those in need cannot pay the fee then the facility is not economically accessible. Accessibility also includes the right to seek, receive and impart information on health. This latter component of accessibility is particularly important for accountability. Protection and enforcement of the right to seek, receive and impart information on health is a prerequisite for accountability. Without publicly available health information, monitoring – an essential element of accountability – will be difficult to undertake.

Regarding acceptability, health facilities must be respectful of medical ethics, be culturally appropriate and gender sensitive. For example, medical treatment must be explained in a manner that is understandable to the person who is to receive the treatment. Health workers will need to be aware of cultural sensitivities in the provision of healthcare – for example, modes of delivery differ according to culture. A gender perspective may need to be incorporated into local health facility budgets to identify gender-based gaps in the budget allocation to health facility programmes. In terms of quality, health facilities must also be scientifically and medically appropriate and of good quality. For example, the provision of a mammography machine to a health centre may not be scientifically and medically appropriate in a situation where resources (human and technical) are scarce and the main health issue for women is HIV. Further, the underlying determinants of health, for example, water and health education, must be appropriate and of good quality too.

Respect, protect and fulfil

The state has specific obligations under international law to respect, protect and fulfil the right to health (General Comment No. 14 2000, paras. 34–7). For example, the obligation to *respect* places an obligation on states to refrain from denying or limiting equal access for all persons (e.g. prisoners, asylum seekers) to health services. The obligation to *protect* means that states should take steps to prevent third parties from jeopardizing the health of others; the private delivery of health services does not nullify government obligation to regulate those services. The obligation to *fulfil* requires governments to adopt necessary measures, including legislative, administrative and budgetary measures, to ensure the full realisation of the right to the highest attainable standard of health (e.g. access to primary healthcare facilities).

iii. Non-discrimination and equality

Central to the right to the highest attainable standard of health is *non-discrimination and equality* (General Comment No. 14, 2000, paras. 18, 19). The right to health belongs to everyone. A person's chances of enjoying good health must not be disadvantaged because of their sex, race, age, language, disability, health status (e.g. with regard to HIV/AIDS), sexual orientation, socioeconomic status, etc. In addition, health policy must be developed in a manner that respects cultural diversity. Special attention must be paid to promoting the equality of disadvantaged groups and gender equality. Indeed, careful consideration of health resource allocations is required to ensure that health policy and spending promote equality rather than perpetuating inequalities, and this is why gender budget analysis is important.

Participation

A further important aspect of the right to health 'is the *participation* of the population in all health-related decision-making at the community, national and international levels'(General Comment No. 14, 2000, para. 11). People are entitled to participate in decision-making and policy formulation relating to their health at local, national and international levels. Steps must be taken to develop mechanisms to enable widespread participation. Importantly, effective participation relies in part upon other rights, such as the right to seek, receive and impart health-related information, the right to express views freely, and the right to basic health education. Full participation on a non-discriminatory basis also requires special attention to sharing information with, and seeking the views of, women and men, as well as the views of disadvantaged people. Participation is essential to the establishment of effective, accessible and easily understood accountability in the context of the right to the highest attainable standard of health.

International assistance and cooperation

In accordance with the obligations envisaged in the United Nations Charter and some human rights treaties, for example the ICESCR, article 2 and the Children's Convention, article 2, less developed countries have a responsibility to seek international assistance and cooperation, while developed countries have some responsibilities towards the realisation of the right to health in less developed countries.

Accountability

As well as the elements set out above, the right to health empowers rights holders to demand accountability. Rights holders are entitled to have access to effective accountability mechanisms at the national, regional (if available) and international levels. National ombudsmen, human rights commissions, consumer forums, patients' rights associations or similar institutions should address violations of the right to health. Rights holders are also entitled to effective remedies when government has failed to discharge its right-to-health obligations. These remedies may take the form of restitution, rehabilitation, compensation, satisfaction or guarantees of non-repetition (General Comment No. 14, 2000, para. 59).

These 10 key elements of the right to health underscore what the right to health contributes to the health sector and to health policy-making. For example, the focus on participation requires a state to adopt an institutional framework that facilitates – to the greatest extent possible – a 'bottom-up' participatory approach. The requirement for monitoring of progressive realisation through indicators will provide the information required for government to identify what is working, what is not and what needs to change. The requirements for accountability mechanisms can help to ensure that health policies are meaningful to those at whom the health policy is directed.

Importantly, the key elements are not to be followed merely because they accord with good health sector management, social justice or ethics. States that are parties to the international and regional human rights treaties that directly or indirectly include the right to health are required to conform to the key features as a matter of international human rights law. Moreover, they are to be held to account for the discharge of their right-to-health obligations arising from these legal obligations.

Accountability

Accountability is a central element of the right to health. While the concept of accountability has preoccupied theorists and researchers in political science and development studies (Newell and Wheeler 2006; Goetz and Jenkins 2005; Darrow and Tomas 2005; Schedler, Diamond and Plattner 1999), little work has been done to identify the component parts of accountability in the context of the right to health generally.[5] It is the identification of these component parts that is the concern of this section.

As a concept, accountability is not new to the health sector (Brinkerhoff 2003). Sometimes it is understood simply in terms of financial accountability: a device to check that health funds are being spent as they should be. At other times, it relates to the performance of the health sector: demonstrating and accounting for performance in light of agreed indicators. It is also understood in a political sense: the presence of institutions, procedures and mechanisms to ensure that the government delivers on its electoral promises, represents citizens' interests, and responds to societal needs and concerns (ibid.: 6–8). It has also been described in terms of a 'short route to accountability', where it is understood as increasing the power of civil society to demand better services from private provision (World Bank 2004: 6).

Right-to-health accountability is also concerned with these categories, but right-to-health accountability is much broader. Accountability in the context of the right to health is the process that provides individuals and communities with an opportunity to understand how government (and its agents) has discharged its right-to-health obligations. Equally, it provides government (and its agents) with the opportunity to explain what it has done and why. Where mistakes have been made, accountability requires redress. It is a process that helps to identify what works, so it can be repeated, and what does not, so it can be revised (Hunt 2008: 23).

Accountability is both prospective and retrospective. Viewed as a prospective process, it draws attention to the potential of accountability to improve performance: to identify what works, so it can be repeated, and what does not, so it can be revised. Viewed as a retrospective process, it draws attention to the remedies that should be available when there has been failure on the part of government to fulfil its obligations. As both a prospective and retrospective process, it necessarily includes the monitoring of conduct, performance and outcomes. It is also continuous (see Figure 3.1 below) and commences with the government ensuring the incorporation and implementation of accountability processes and procedures into all health policy.

The accountability process requires the incorporation of monitoring into all aspects of policy development and implementation. This monitoring is conducted by government on a continuous basis. It can also be conducted by civil society, either collaboratively with government, independently, or both. The accountability processes and procedures also require the presence of accessible accountability mechanisms to provide a forum for explanation and justification. This explanation and justification can take place in a variety of settings, and need not be confined to formal settings such as the courts or national human rights institutions (NHRIs). Other settings include democratically elected health councils, public hearings and national or local public meetings; the media also has a crucial role to play. In addition, remedies for the non-fulfilment of right-to-health obligations are to be available. Remedies, in the context of the right to health, are broad in nature as they include

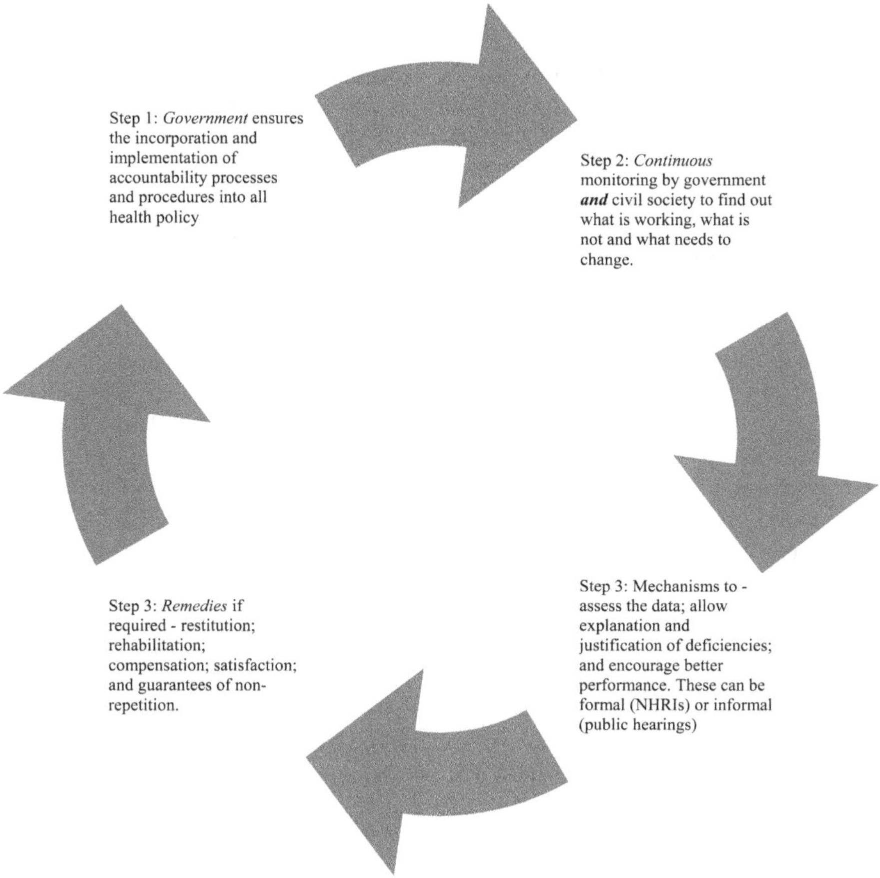

Figure 3.1 The Accountability Process

modification of monitoring processes, inclusion of human rights training, and organisational improvements concerning planning, budgeting and policy formulation, in addition to judicial remedies such as compensation. Participation is present in each of these elements – monitoring, mechanisms and remedies. While the form of participation will vary, for example, between accountability mechanisms (judicial vs. social) it is an essential element of accountability. An effective accountability process is therefore comprised of the following essential elements: monitoring, mechanisms, remedies and participation.

Accountability is not the same as responsiveness, responsibility, answerability or evaluation, as none of these concepts include a legal compulsion to explain and to provide remedies; meaningful accountability is not possible without monitoring. Progressively realising the right to health requires that policies and practice be brought into line with right-to-health standards. Monitoring must therefore be able to indicate what is working, what is not working, what has been omitted and what changes need to be made. Monitoring plays a dual role in relation to accountability: (i) it provides, on an ongoing basis, the information that government needs to determine what areas should be focused on in order to reach its targets for the realisation of the right to health; and (ii) it provides rights holders with the information they need to claim their rights and to hold the government and its agents to account when obligations have not been fulfilled.

Health policy-makers use a very large number of health indicators that are relevant to health policy effectiveness and national and international reporting. However, these health indicators do not usually capture all that right to health monitoring demands. For example, right to health monitoring would also require indicators on the participation of individuals and groups in the development, implementation and review of health policy, as well as indicators on the protection of the right to seek, receive and impart information on the right to health. Ways to address this important deficiency in health indicators can be found elsewhere, for example, in the report of the Special Rapporteur on the right to health, submitted to the Commission on Human Rights in 2006 (Hunt 2006: 12–14).

As rights holders are entitled to obtain information and as government has an obligation to release all relevant material, the results of monitoring must be made public. When the findings are released, they are an important tool for accountability. There are multiple avenues available to government for the release of this information. For example, in many countries there is an institution at the national level that reports on the health status of a population on a periodic basis. Right-to-health monitoring information could be included in these reports. In addition, many countries have a national human rights plan. The information gained from monitoring could also be released in the annual report to parliament on the implementation of the national human rights plan. This monitoring information could also be made available at the regional and international levels.

Government has an obligation to monitor its own activity. In addition, government activity must also be monitored by civil society. Too much dependency on government monitoring could result in unquestioningly accepting the data that is offered. Accordingly, as part of the right to seek, receive and impart information, civil society organisations should perform a monitoring role. This monitoring role can be undertaken independently or in cooperation with the government and its agents.

In India, for example, the Jan Swasthya Abhiyan (JSA or People's Health Movement – India) has had an ongoing process of critical engagement with the National Rural Health Mission (NRHM) framework in the form of the People's Rural Health Watch (PRHW). The PRHW is an independent initiative by JSA to audit the state of rural public health services periodically, particularly in the light of the official NRHM initiative. This auditing is independent of the official framework and has been conceptualised and implemented entirely by the JSA. This programme has been implemented in seven northern states and involves JSA member organisations independently collecting information about the activities conducted under the NHRM, both at the state and national levels (Potts 2008: 16).[6]

The above examples, as relevant to the North as they are to the South, highlight that health policy makers need to be aware of how civil society monitoring can assist them in their work and how they can work cooperatively with civil society to progressively implement the right to health and ensure government accountability for its implementation.

Accountability mechanisms

An accountability mechanism is the procedure through which government is answerable for its acts or omissions in relation to right-to-health obligations. The procedure provides rights holders with an opportunity to obtain information on government action and ask for explanations. It also provides government with an opportunity to explain its actions. In the absence of accessible and effective accountability mechanisms, the right to health will be largely meaningless to rights holders.

Broadly speaking, there are five types of accountability mechanisms: judicial, quasi-judicial, administrative, political and social. Space does not permit a detailed explanation of each of these mechanisms together with examples of 'accountability in action'. Accordingly, a short description of each is provided.[7] First, judicial: the entrenchment of the right to health, either directly or indirectly, in the national constitution (or other legislation) may provide a specific right-to-health accountability mechanism which can provide access to the courts to enable rights holders to challenge government legislation and policy. See for example the Minister of Health vs. Treatment Action Campaign (TAC Case) which concerned State provisions of nevirapine, an antiretroviral drug used to prevent mother-to-child transmission (MTCT) of HIV. The Constitutional Court confirmed that the Government must act reasonably to provide access to the socioeconomic rights contained in the Constitution. The Court ordered the Government to develop a reasonable policy for this purpose, that is, one that was comprehensive and co-ordinated between all levels of government, and which focussed upon those in need – in this case, pregnant women and their new-born children who had been effectively denied access to the drug. Judicial mechanisms can also hold government to account through the identification of legislation which is inconsistent with international human rights obligations, judicial review of executive decision-making, statutory interpretation and the review of administrative tribunal decision-making.

Second, in regards to quasi-judicial measures, NHRIs can be described in broad terms as independent bodies established by government for the specific purpose of advancing and defending human rights (Pohjolainen 2006: 1). NHRIs can take many forms, and range from human rights commissions to human rights ombudsperson and public defenders. NHRIs frequently work with social accountability mechanisms to ensure the implementation of the right to health and government accountability. In addition, general quasi-judicial bodies such as patients' rights commissions or tribunals, healthcare commissions and health complaints tribunals are present in many countries. They are usually autonomous bodies created pursuant to legislation. The mandate and powers of these quasi-judicial bodies varies, and can include determining complaints about the public health service, the independent health service and health workers. They can also carry out reviews of public and independent health sector performance, and investigations and research into the public health sector. Their focus tends to be on the curative health sector rather than underlying determinants or prevention. Nevertheless, their work provides important assistance regarding the right to health for health policy makers through the issues they identify, the decisions of the tribunals, and the findings and recommendations of research and investigations.

In regards to the third type of accountability mechanism, administrative, the human rights impact assessment (HRIA) is a relatively recent concept that seeks to predict the potential consequences of a proposed policy on the enjoyment of human rights (Hunt and MacNaughton 2006). The objective of HRIA is to introduce an explicit process into the existing repertoire of actions undertaken by decision-makers or groups of people likely to be affected by decision-making so that they can take action to improve the policy before it is implemented. The process seeks, to reduce potential negative impacts on the population, and to enhance the potential positive impacts of a proposed action.

The development of HRIA provides some useful guiding points which could be used to underpin HRIA particularly the work completed on the production of the equity-focused health impact assessment framework (EFHIA) (Mahoney *et al.* 2004). Both forms of impact assessment are concerned with ensuring that the concerns of the most vulnerable and marginalised people in the population are included in the policy-making process in more explicit ways. Just as HRIA is concerned with ensuring the meaningful participation of people in decisions that affect their lives and without discrimination, EFHIA emphasises the right of people to participate in decisions that affect them and identify the distribution of the impact of a policy within the population.

The fourth mechanism, political accountability, depends on the nature of the political system in a country, and hence the power of a political accountability mechanism, will vary from one country to another. Despite this variation, political accountability is central. Through linkages to social accountability mechanisms, especially the media, political accountability can ensure effective remedies, particularly those of *satisfaction and guarantees of non-repetition*. Included within political accountability mechanisms are parliamentary committees, health councils, and free and fair elections.

Parliamentary committees exist in many countries and they come in almost endless varieties (Mattson and Strom 1995; Caesar-Katsenga and Myburg 2006). They can be either specific or general accountability mechanisms; their function and composition varies from country to country. They conduct inquiries into specified matters such as investigation of policy issues, proposed legislation or government activities such as international assistance and cooperation. During this process, they may take submissions and hear witnesses. Accordingly, this accountability mechanism can also provide a forum for a form of participation by civil society. Although the parliamentary committee process provides an important accountability mechanism, it is a mechanism that is weak in many countries, and therefore requires capacity building. Health councils represent a form of political accountability that has gained considerable popularity in recent decades. Usually statutory bodies, they are present in many countries and have a variety of powers (though not always, as they can be created through policy). Their powers vary, from the approval of health plans and budgets, to the provision of a complaints mechanism (in which case they overlap with quasi-judicial mechanisms), to simply attempting to increase the voice of civil society in the development of health policy.

Free and fair elections can provide a retrospective general accountability mechanism through removing governments from office for failure to implement electoral promises. It is a generally agreed assumption that free and fair elections by themselves are no guarantee of good governance (Newell 2006: 42; Goetz and Jenkins 2005: 18–20). While they provide a means of accountability of government to citizens, they occur only periodically and their accountability can be unclear in the presence of poorly defined issues and sudden policy reversals (O'Donnell 1998: 113).

Fifth, social accountability mechanisms involve citizen action to oversee government conduct. Through a process of social mobilisation and the use of the media, these mechanisms can provide a set of checks and balances on the proper conduct of government (Newell 2006: 47–8). Social accountability mechanisms can act as quasi-official agents, either participating directly in accountability mechanisms or substituting for failing state accountability institutions. They regularly work with other accountability mechanisms, for example quasi-judicial mechanisms, to obtain a response from government and to monitor government accountability processes.

Social accountability mechanisms can also create new formal accountability mechanisms, for example the development of the NGO Shadow Report to the United Nations treaty monitoring bodies such as the Committee on Economic, Social and Cultural Rights and the Committee on the Elimination of All Forms of Discrimination Against Women. There are myriad national, regional and international civil society movements working individually and collaboratively to develop mechanisms to call governments to account for implementation of the right to health.

The media also plays a significant role in today's society by providing a very wide range of information in a variety of ways. The media strongly influences community attitudes, beliefs and behaviour, plays a vital role in politics, economics and social practice, and can influence political popularity. Civil society movements frequently engage the media and hence rely on the presence of a free media that is willing to engage in critical journalism.[8] The effectiveness of social accountability mechanisms is weakened in the absence of the protection and enforcement of the human rights of expression, association and information.

Effective remedies

Remedies to redress violations of the right to health are key to ensuring that human rights have meaning. *All* of the remedies mentioned below should be available through the judicial accountability mechanism of every state that is a party to the ICESCR. Many of these remedies, for example full and public disclosure of the truth, or renewed commitment to an original obligation, or inclusion of right-to-health training for government and health workers, could also be made available through other accountability mechanisms, in particular the quasi-judicial and political mechanisms. In addition, remedies such as apologies or the introduction of right-to-health training could be made available within social accountability mechanisms such as public hearings and mass social audits.

Remedies may take any one or more of the following forms: (i) restitution; (ii) compensation; (iii) rehabilitation; or (iv) satisfaction. Restitution involves the re-establishment of a situation that existed prior to the violation of the right to health. For example, if legislation or policy has been introduced to limit access to healthcare services by particular groups, restitution would involve either amendment of the legislation or reversal of the policy. Compensation should be provided for any economically assessable damage resulting from a violation of human rights. The state has an obligation to take all necessary measures to safeguard persons within their jurisdiction from infringements of the right to health by third parties. For example, illness and injury caused through the non-regulation of privately controlled industries resulting in chemical contamination of air and water. Economically assessable damage includes:

- physical or mental harm, including pain, suffering and emotional distress;
- loss of opportunity, for example, education;
- costs required for medicines and medical services;
- material damages and loss of earnings, including future economic loss; and
- costs required for legal or expert assistance.

Rehabilitation includes medical and psychological care as well as legal and social services. As rehabilitation includes provision of social services, this remedy could include the provision services such as the provision of water and basis sanitation. The final remedies – satisfaction, and guarantees of non-repetition include:

- a full and public disclosure of the truth;
- an apology, including public acknowledgement of the facts and acceptance of responsibility;
- an official declaration or a judicial decision;

- a judicial or administrative sanctions against the persons responsible for the violations;
- the inclusion of right-to-health training for government and health workers;
- the conduct of right-to-health training to all sectors of society, in particular to government ministers and their department staff and members of other political parties;
- legislation;
- monitoring and enforcement mechanisms;
- organisational improvements in the ministry concerning planning, budgeting, policy formulation; and
- a renewed commitment to, or reaffirmation of, the original obligation accompanied by an action plan including benchmarks and dates for achievement.

The first three remedies focus on the rights holder and are concerned with redressing the impact of the violation of the individual or group rights holder. The last remedies – satisfaction, and guarantees of non-repetition – are particularly important in ensuring the introduction of accountability mechanisms in the long term.

Conclusion

The previous sections have aimed to provide an introductory picture to accountability in the context of the right to health. It is by no means the end of the story. Investigation into the concept of accountability and the right to health is a relatively new area: much more needs to be done to further refine the concept. For example, the application of the elements of accountability to specific issues, such as HIV/AIDS, would be one way of further refining accountability in the context of the right to the highest attainable standard of health.

Though there remains much to be done, it is possible to provide the following list of pre-conditions for effective accountability:

- A strong commitment and long-term vision on the part of government that the right to health should be incorporated into the day-to-day work of health policy-makers;
- the presence of a national health plan that incorporates the right to health;
- institutional mechanisms to ensure effective participation in the development, implementation and review of the national health plan;
- the establishment of effective institutional arrangements for civil society and the government to work together;
- the establishment of effective monitoring systems;
- access to, and implementation of, the decisions of accountability mechanisms that are relevant to health policy; and
- the development of ongoing right to health training for health policy makers at all levels.

Notes

1 This paper draws upon the monograph Potts, H. (2008) *Accountability and the right to the highest attainable standard of health*, University of Essex: Human Rights Centre. Online. Available http://www2.essex.ac.uk/human_rights_centre/rth/projects.shtm (accessed 13 August 2008). The monograph was developed by Doctor Helen Potts, when a Senior Researcher Officer to Professor Paul Hunt, United Nations Special Rapporteur on the right of everyone to the enjoyment of the highest attainable standard of physical and Mental Health (August 2002–July 2008). The research was supported by a grant from the Open Society Institute. As part of the consultation process, a draft of the monograph was presented at the CSGR/UNDP conference 'Governance of HIV/AIDS Response: Making participation and accountability count' held at the University of Warwick, 5–6 November 2007.

2 This framework is applied throughout the work of Professor Paul Hunt, when Special Rapporteur on the right of everyone to the enjoyment of the highest attainable standard of physical and mental health. Online: http://www2.essex.ac.uk/human_rights_centre/rth/reports.shtm (accessed 25 August 2008).

3 See for example the Participation and Practice of Rights Project, Belfast where the residents of the Seven Towers block have developed a set of indicators for the monitoring of the obligations of the Northern Ireland Housing Executive. Online. Available http://www.pprproject.org/ (accessed 13 August 2008).

4 The Committee on Economic, Social and Cultural Rights defined 'health facilities, goods and services' in *General Comment No. 14*, to include the underlying determinants of health as outlined in paragraphs 11 and 12(a) of the General Comment. For convenience, the term 'health facilities' will be used throughout the remainder of this paper.

5 This is not to say that no work has been done. See for example, Yamin, A (2005) "The Future in the Mirror: Incorporating Strategies for the Defense and Promotion of Economic, Social and Cultural rights into the Mainstream Human Rights Agenda", *Human Rights Quarterly* 27:1200; Murthy, R. Klugman, B. and Weller, S. (with contributions from Aizenberg, L.) (2005) "Service Accountability and Community Participation" in T.K.S Ravindran and H. (eds) *The Right Reforms? Health Sector Reforms and Sexual and Reproductive Health*, Parktown S.A.: Women's Health Project; Freedman, L. (2003) "Human rights, constructive accountability and maternal mortality in the Dominican Republic: a commentary", *International Journal of Gynecology and Obstetrics*, 82: 111.

6 See also the publication *Dignity Counts: A Guide to Using Budget Analysis to Advance Human Rights.* This publication, prepared by *Fundar-Centro de Análisis e Investigación*, the International Budget Project and the International Human Rights Internship Program, draws upon a case study of the Mexican national government budget to provide guidance to civil society organisations and others on how to use budget analysis as a tool to assess government compliance regarding economic, social and cultural rights obligations.

7 Greater detail on the examples is given in the monograph *Accountability and the right to the highest attainable standard of health*, referred to above in note I, pages 17–27.

8 For an excellent description of how social accountability mechanism engage the media see Heywood, M. 'Preventing Mother-to-Child HIV Transmission in South Africa: Background, Strategies and Outcomes of the Treatment Action Campaign Case against the Minister of Health' (2003) 19 *South African Journal of Human Rights* 278–315. See also the NGO Women's Link Worldwide and the video on the liberalisation of abortion in Colombia. Online: http://www.womenslinkworldwide.org/ (accessed 29 August 2008).

Bibliography

Brinkerhoff, D. (2003). *Accountability and Health Systems: Overview, Framework, and Strategies.* Technical Report No. 018. January. Bethesda, MD: The Partners for Health Reform*plus* Project, Abt Associates Inc.

Caesar-Katsenga, M. and Myburg, M. (2006) *Parliaments, Politics and HIV/AIDS: A comparative study of five African countries*, Pretoria/Cape Town: Idasa. Online. http://www.idasa.org.za/ (accessed 26 August 2008).

Committee on Economic, Social and Cultural Rights, *General Comment No. 14: The right to the highest attainable standard of health* (2000) UN Doc E/C.12/2000/4. Online. http://www2.ohchr.org/english/bodies/cescr/comments.htm (accessed 29 August 2008).

Convention on the Rights of the Child, adopted and opened for signature, ratification and accession by General Assembly Resolution 44/25 of 20 November 1989, 1577 UNTS 3 (entered into force 2 September 1990). Online. http://www2.ohchr.org/english/law/index.htm#core (accessed 26 August 2008).

Darrow, M. and Tomas, A. (2005). 'Power, Capture, and Conflict: A Call for Human Rights Accountability in Development Cooperation', *Human Rights Quarterly*, 27: 471.

Fundar, International Human Rights Internship Program, International Budget Project. (2004). *Dignity Counts: A guide to using budget analysis to advance human rights*, Online. http://www.iie.org/IHRIP/Dignity_Counts.pdf (accessed 29 August 2008).

Goetz, A. and Jenkins, R. (2005). *Reinventing Accountability: Making Democracy Work for Human Development*, New York: Palgrave Macmillan.

Hunt, P. (2006). *Report of the Special Rapporteur on the Right of Everyone to the Enjoyment of the Highest Attainable Standard of Physical and Mental Health* UN Doc. E/CN.4/2006/48, 3 March 2006. Online. http://www2.essex.ac.uk/human_rights_centre/rth/reports.shtm (accessed 29 August 2008).

Hunt, P. (2008). *Report of the Special Rapporteur on the Right of Everyone to the Enjoyment of the Highest Attainable Standard of Physical and Mental Health* UN Doc. A/HRC/7/11, 31 January 2008. Online. http://www2.essex.ac.uk/human_rights_centre/rth/docs/A-HRC-7–11.doc (accessed 26 August 2008).

Hunt, P. and MacNaughton, G. (2006) *Impact Assessments, Poverty and Human Rights: A Case Study Using The Right to the Highest Attainable Standard of Health.* Online. http://www2.essex.ac.uk/human_rights_centre/rth/projects.shtm (accessed 29 August 2008).

International Covenant on Economic, Social and Cultural Rights, opened for signature 19th December 1966, 993 UNTS 3 (entered into force 3rd January 1976).

Kinney, E. and Clark, B. (2004). 'Provisions for Health and Healthcare in the Constitutions of the Countries of the World', *Cornell International Law Journal*, 37: 285.

Mahoney, M. Simpson, S. Harris, E. Aldrich, R. and Stewart Williams, J. (2004). *Equity-Focused Health Impact Assessment Framework*, Melbourne: Australasian Collaboration for Health Equity Impact Assessment. Online. http://www.deakin.edu.au/hmnbs/hia/publications.php (accessed 29 August 2008).

Mattson, I. and Strom, K. (1995). 'Parliamentary Committees' in H. Döring (ed.) *Parliaments and Majority Rule in Western Europe*, Frankfurt/NewYork: Campus Verlag, St. Martin.

Newell, P. (2006) 'Taking accountability into account: the debate so far', in P. Newell and J. Wheeler (eds) *Rights, Resources and the Politics of Accountability*, London: Zed Books.

Newell, P. and Wheeler, J. (eds) (2006). *Rights, Resources and the Politics of Accountability*, London: Zed Books.

Minister of Health v Treatment Action Campaign (2002). CCT 8/02.

O'Donnell, G. (1998). 'Horizontal Accountability in New Democracies' *Journal of Democracy*, 9: 112–26.

Paschim Banga Khet Mazdoor Samity and Ors v State of West Bengal 1996(4) SCC 37.

Pohjolainen, A. (2006). *The Evolution of National Human Rights Institutions. The Role of the United Nations.* Copenhagen: Danish Institute for Human Rights. Online: http://www.foerderverein-mri.ch/c_data/Evolution_of_NHRIs.pdf (accessed 29 August 2008).

Potts, H. (2008). *Accountability and the right to the highest attainable standard of health*, University of Essex: Human Rights Centre. Online. http://www2.essex.ac.uk/human_rights_centre/rth/projects.shtm (accessed 13 August 2008).

Schedler, A. Diamond L. and Plattner, M. (1999). *The Self-Restraining State: Power and Accountability in New Democracies*, London: Lynne Rienner Publishers.

The International Bank for Reconstruction and Development/The World Bank. (2003). *World Development Report 2004: Making Health Services Work for the Poor*, Washington: World Bank and Oxford University Press. Online. http://www.worldbank.org (accessed 26 August 2008).

4 The Home-Based Care Alliance in Kenya

Improving governance and transforming communities in the context of HIV/AIDS

Shannon Hayes[1]

> So many people know that the CACC is ineffective, but they had no way to address these issues. So we thought if we could find a way to mobilize the community to come together and discuss this, that would be a good idea … (the CACC members) now look at us like people who know.
>
> Violet Shivutse, founder of the Kakamega District Home-Based Care Alliance

Understandings of HIV/AIDS governance have thus far focussed upon the role of international organisations, the state and the operations and effectiveness of national AIDS councils from the perspective of national government and international funding. It is widely accepted that HIV/AIDS has most severely affected people in poor and marginalised communities, and the scale of grassroots contributions to mitigating the effects of HIV/AIDS is increasingly well documented and understood; the realities, capacities and priorities of community practitioners are regularly excluded, however. Moreover, a gap exists between the mandates and intentions of national AIDS councils and the realities facing communities affected by and coping with HIV/AIDS. Through a case study detailing the community response to HIV/AIDS led by an organised group of home-based caregivers, this chapter offers a model for closing this gap between intention and reality, and investigates how alternative funding mechanisms might function.

Where investments of resources and time have been made in organisation and leadership development, organised groups of grassroots women have been able to use the urgency created by the AIDS epidemic to strengthen the position of women within local level decision-making and resource allocation structures – women who are generally marginalised and excluded from such institutional processes. The unprecedented devastation caused by the AIDS pandemic, and the spotlight it has shined on poverty and gender inequality in Sub-Saharan Africa, has created international political will and mobilised significant resources that are in turn creating unique opportunities for grassroots women's organisations to build women's empowerment, strengthen their constituencies and promote good governance, accountability and transparency. While there are multiple complex challenges associated with the decentralised funding structures that have been established in countries like Kenya, this chapter will demonstrate that these can be overcome through direct support for grassroots women-led initiatives. Where investments have been made in grassroots women-led organisation, women have been able to build partnerships with local government, thereby improving governance processes, accountability, transparency and service delivery.

The chapter proceeds in the following manner. First, it provides an overview of the AIDS epidemic in Kenya and the response to the epidemic both by the government of Kenya and by home-based caregivers, setting the context for our case study. Second, through a case study the chapter will demonstrate that home-based caregivers are uniquely positioned to improve the governance of AIDS structures starting at the local level through facilitating dialogues between communities and the councils and governmental structures charged with responding to AIDS. The chapter concludes with a set of recommendations based on the lessons learned in the case study, arguing that investments need to be made in organising and building the capacity of women to engage in structures, and local AIDS authorities need to be pushed to establish permanent mechanisms to involve organised groups of citizens.

This chapter argues that the process of decentralised funding and political responsibility within the global response to HIV/AIDS is creating a unique opportunity to create partnerships between civil society and local government to build good governance, accountability and transparency. The creation of these decentralised mechanisms has been vital in bringing funding and decision-making power to where the government meets the community. However, the structures and mechanisms are in many cases highly politicised, and suffer from a lack of technical, financial and infrastructural resources, which impedes the delivery of much-needed resources and services to those infected.

In this chapter, we use the terms effectiveness and accountability from the perspective of grassroots communities. Funds are effective when they get to the people, organisations and institutions that are providing sustainable, ongoing interventions to HIV and AIDS that are responsive to the immediate and long-term needs of communities. Structures are accountable when they are in communication with, open to and responsive to, the needs of those communities. The main findings of the chapter are drawn from the experiences of the Home-Based Care Alliance in Kenya. We have chosen to focus on Kenya for three reasons. The first is our desire to illustrate a limited, national example of how decision-making processes are functioning in the context of AIDS. Second, Kenya is a country that is undergoing a conscious movement to strengthen democracy following a long period of one-man rule. Third, we have in Kenya a powerful example of grassroots women organising for greater participation, and federating across communities and regions to build power and share and analyse the lessons. Civil society is generally recognized as one key part of a strong multi-stakeholder response to AIDS. Civil society in the form of a professional non-governmental organisation (NGO) is not necessarily well placed to build good governance or accountability, however, as those NGOs tend to be accountable to their board or donors rather than the populations that they serve. Civil society organisations in this chapter refer to self-organised groups of citizens living and working in their own communities, in this case a group of home-based caregivers. Their efforts are aimed at building the capacity of their communities to participate in the structures that were designed to include them and to hold accountable the institutions and actors who are supposed to be accountable to them.

Context: The AIDS epidemic and the global response

According to the AIDS Epidemic Update of 2004, 39.5 million people are currently infected by HIV. AIDS is a global pandemic, which is taking its worst toll in the poorest regions of the world. More than 60 per cent of all adults and 76 per cent of all women infected with HIV worldwide live in Sub-Saharan Africa. In Kenya alone, where the latest estimates place the adult prevalence rate at 6.1 per cent, almost 500 people per day are dying of AIDS and life expectancy is 47 years, down from 53 in 1975. New infections are occurring daily, mostly among young people and women (UNAIDS/WHO 2004).

UNAIDS notes the dual impact of the AIDS epidemic – upon families and upon countries. Families feel the immediate impact of losing the primary breadwinner; communities and nations feel the gradual of losing a large percentage of breadwinners. Not only are countries with large HIV-positive infections made poorer by AIDS, they are also left more vulnerable to its impact by the fact that they are already marginalised in the global economy because they had few resources to deal with the disease at its start. Structural adjustment programs of the 1980s and 90s left most African countries even more vulnerable, with government per capita expenditure on health care as a percentage of GDP falling from 7 per cent in the 1970s to 2 per cent today. (Oyaya and Rifkin 2003; Earth Trends 2003).

Academic research supports the double tie of AIDS to development – with poverty as both cause and consequence of the disease. Poverty, industrialisation, and the associated breakdown of traditional modes of employment and interpersonal relations and support systems, have left communities vulnerable to AIDS. Poverty, food insecurity and resultant malnutrition, and job insecurity are all factors in the spread of HIV, and dependency development and economic decline set the larger context for the creation of an epidemic driven by poverty (Whiteside 2002; Gordon 1995; Hunt 1989). The UN has cited HIV/AIDS as one of the largest single obstacles to meeting the Millennium Development Goals (United Nations 2001).

In Kenya, an estimated 1.3 million adults (roughly 7 per cent of the adult population) and 50–100,000 children are currently living with HIV in Kenya. AIDS kills approximately 150,000 people a year, and there are currently about 1 million orphans. As is the case elsewhere on the continent, women are disproportionately affected, accounting for about 60 per cent of the HIV-positive population, and nearly two-thirds of HIV-positive people in Kenya are women (UNAIDS/WHO 2004). The reasons for the increasing feminisation of AIDS are biological – in that women are simply more vulnerable to contracting the virus – sociocultural and economic. High levels of polygamy and widely practiced extramarital sex have also been factors in the rapid spread of HIV throughout Sub-Saharan Africa (Caldwell 2000). Women and children are left more vulnerable by widespread practice of disinheritance (Strickland 2004). The lack of opportunities for paid work, due to high rates of poverty and unemployment in Kenya, enhances high-risk behaviour among unmarried women (Hunt 1989).

A decentralised response to AIDS

As knowledge of the scale and impact of HIV/AIDS emerged throughout the 1990s, the World Bank, UN and other development agencies encouraged and supported national governments in Sub-Saharan Africa to establish national AIDS councils in order to develop national AIDS policies, spearhead advocacy, build partnerships and lead resource mobilisation, among other functions.[2] These AIDS councils have largely been established along decentralised lines. It seems that AIDS is a global problem that the global development community has rightly decided is best solved through a wide range of community-centered micro-solutions.

In response to the epidemic in Kenya, the government established a national AIDS council with financial and technical support from the World Bank's Multi-Country AIDS Programme. To date, the World Bank and the Global Fund for AIDS, Tuberculosis and Malaria (Global Fund) have transferred US$348,897,067 to the Government of Kenya for fighting AIDS.[3] The Kenyan National AIDS Control Council (NACC) is responsible for the implementation of the Kenya National Strategic AIDS Plan and its decentralised agencies – district and provincial aids control committees – which coordinate the response in their respective locations. The Constituency AIDS Control Committees (CACCs) are responsible for the coordination of efforts at the community level, and are also grant-making bodies, authorised by arliament to fund community-driven responses to AIDS. This decentralised structure was established with the intent to ensure that monies for AIDS responses were reaching the community level; that multiple stakeholders, including those representing community priorities, were involved in defining national AIDS policy, and a strong response was being coordinated at the community level where it was most needed. (World Bank 2000; UNAIDS/WHO 2004). The structure of the Kenyan NACC, relationships between its constituent parts and relative responsibilities are described in diagram 4.1.

Decentralisation and governance

The decentralised model of AIDS structures fit in with a wider rationale of decentralisation in government. Because AIDS structures are built along a decentralised model, it is informative at this point to draw parallels between

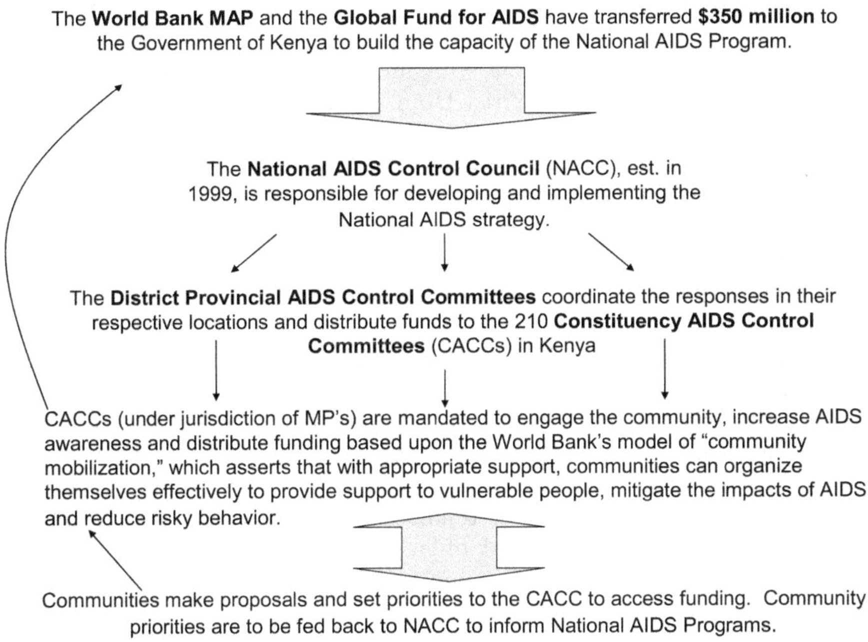

Diagram 4.1 The Kenya National AIDS Control Council structure (World Bank 2000)

decentralisation in government and the NACC/CACC system. A decentralised system is supposed to foster greater accountability, transparency and participation – and hence democracy – thus decision-making takes place at the level of government closest to the people – generally under the mayor or local authority. Justification for decentralisation is closely associated with the emphasis placed on good governance by the international development community. Governance in this sense is defined by the UN as:

> The exercise of economic, political and administrative authority to manage a country's affairs at all levels. It comprises the mechanisms, processes and institutions through which citizens and groups articulate their interests, exercise their legal rights, meet their obligations and mediate their differences.
>
> (NRC 2003)

If governance defines the relationship between governed and governors, *good* governance implies decision-making processes that are inclusive, participatory, accountable, transparent and with an emphasis on process. Good governance also assumes the active involvement of civil society organisations (CSOs). Local-level engagement with, and promotion of, civil society can also, it is assumed, become a platform for the promotion of greater democracy at the local level.

Decentralisation has also come with many challenges which we will see echoed in by the Kakamega District Home-Based Care Alliance. First, there is evidence that, without mandatory participatory structures, decentralisation leads to the so-called capture of resources by local elites, thereby reinforcing social inequalities. Decision-making structures will also exclude those who are already marginalised without clear standards of representation. (Hadiz 2003; UNAIDS/WHO 2004; Huairou Commission 2007).

A second impediment to the benefits of decentralisation is low skills and knowledge-based capacity at the local level. The local-level democratic processes, upon which decentralisation are premised, are based upon both the ability of local authorities and council members to deliver the decentralised services, and the capability of the community members to understand the functioning of those structures and their entitlements. Citizens must also be able to understand the new powers and responsibilities being placed into the hands of their communities. Unfortunately, many citizens in poor countries are poorly educated, illiterate and often apathetic – all factors of marginalisation. Civil society, in partnership with governments, is often ideally placed to mitigate these factors and foster greater citizen participation in local-level processes, particularly citizens' groups, such as those that make up the Home-Based Care Alliance. As we will see in the case study, the Kakamega District Home-Based Care Alliance responded to these challenges by bringing together stakeholders from all levels of society in an open meeting, in order to facilitate the community to identify its problems and priorities, and to explain the institutions they were negotiating with.

In addition to these general challenges in decentralisation, there are a number of challenges that have been identified by grassroots organisations or grassroots-focussed NGOs as specific to national AIDS councils (ACTAfrica 2006), these include:

- politicised planning, implementation and funding mechanisms that foster corruption, nepotism and opportunism;
- national structures that do not provide for horizontal participation and accountability;
- irregular information flows from the government to the grassroots level;
- monitoring and evaluation of national AIDS funding structures/mechanisms that do not ensure participation of affected communities;
- grassroots groups' voices being subordinated within the 'civil society' mandate; and
- proposal requirements favouring 'established' NGOs and exclude grassroots organisations who often have limited capacity for writing.

Analyses of the opportunities and challenges presented by the decentralisation of health services in Kenya are also informative here. The reform of the health sector in Kenya began in the late 1980s and resulted in a re-organisation of health services on principles of decentralisation and community participation, with an emphasis on the non-governmental sector (Oyaya and Rifkin 2003). As a part of this process, District Health Management Teams (DHMTs) were established to ensure multi-stakeholder involvement in the health sector at the local level. While the study by Oyaya and Rifkin found that DHMT members found the decentralised system preferable because of the freedom of responsiveness to local concerns it allowed them, they expressed concerns about governance and accountability at the district level. DHMT board members were supposed to be appointed by the Minister of Health based on their standing as people of high respect and technical expertise. However, the reality turned out to be that they were usually appointed based on their political connections and for reasons of patronage. Thus composed, the boards very rarely if ever included poor people or leaders of organised groups of poor people, or consulted poor people for their health priorities. As the study stated, 'community decision-making bodies created to strengthen accountability by giving a "voice" to the community often did not appear to serve the interests of the poorest' (Oyaya and Rifkin 2003) This is the same situation currently being exhibited in the CACCs, which are under the jurisdiction of Parliament.

What communities contribute

According to the general operations manual of the World Bank's MAP, *Turning Bureaucrats into Warriors*:

> The scale of the HIV/AIDS crisis necessitates the fullest possible CSO involvement at all levels. Most people with HIV infection or illness already receive most of their support and care from the community, not from formal institutions. Only through community involvement can programs of sufficient number, scope, coverage and value for resources and effort be achieved. Yet there is discontinuity between formal and informal responses that has not been adequately addressed. Formal responses seldom reach or provide appropriate support to community initiatives and communities are seldom able to access formal support.
>
> (Brown *et al.* 2004: 37)

For grassroots women living and coping with HIV/AIDS, the epidemic is not simply a health issue. Its causes and effects are deeply linked to every aspect of their lives, and grassroots communities know that HIV cannot be addressed without other related issues of development and human settlements. Through home-based care, grassroots women are creating a holistic, women-led, community-driven response to HIV/AIDS. Grassroots women coping with the AIDS pandemic on a daily basis are clear that HIV is not just a health issue. It is an issue encompassing all aspects of daily life – access to basic services including water, sanitation and transportation, livelihoods, food security and governance. Home-based caregivers provide palliative care, treatment for opportunistic infections and psychosocial counselling; they initiate locally appropriate and culturally sensitive stigma-reduction and awareness-raising campaigns, provide nutritional counselling and promote food security. As demonstrated in the case study, they are also improving access to basic services by linking to the existing formal services, including clinics and hospitals, mortuaries, feeding programs, and to resources such as bursary funds for orphans.

While some of the direct health aspects of treating HIV have improved over the past decade, most notably due to access to antiretroviral treatment (ART), the related livelihood and development factors that have made HIV/AIDS so devastating in resource-poor countries, particularly in Africa, have not improved. Grassroots women in organised self-help groups are therefore left to deal with lack of health, transportation, water and sanitation infrastructure, poor economic opportunities and governmental corruption and misallocation of resources, in addition to linking neighbours and relatives to health clinics and hospitals for ART, and monitoring adherence to the drug programmes. Caregivers are also providing wide-ranging family support for HIV-affected families, not just for individuals infected with the virus. As they work in their own communities, with which they are intimately familiar, caregivers gain the trust of the community through their capabilities, discretion and diligence, and are able to reach the most marginalised and isolated cases, providing care, linking them to information and services without necessarily revealing their status to the community.

Understanding of the multi-faceted causes and effects is growing, which is reflected in recent research and programming more directly linking HIV to development, such as the World Health Organisation (WHO)'s campaign on food security, and the International Center for Research on Women's focus on the links between women's land, inheritance and property rights, and AIDS (Strickland 2004; WHO 2007). However, the complex interplay of poverty, culture and women's inequality, which is intrinsically understood by grassroots women working on these issues on the ground, has yet to be fully documented and analysed by researchers, or to have more than a token impact on programme design, policy-making and funding.

There is an immense and unequal burden placed on caregivers – women and girls in particular – and, as acknowledged above, this burden in many cases leaves women more vulnerable to HIV infection as it limits their ability to earn an income. It is clear that there is much work to be done to properly recognise, valorise and compensate the important contributions that home-based caregivers are making. It should be noted that many men also provide home-based care and participate in the Home-Based Care Alliance. Feminist economists in particular have placed a great emphasis on women's unpaid care work and have produced many comprehensive analyses of the care economy (Razavi 2007; Urdang 2006; Mehta and Gupta 2006). Their policy recommendations, however, tend to be aimed at policy-makers and focussed on budgetary increases in the formal health sector and increasing formal training and capacity-building for home-based caregivers, and rarely or insufficiently take into account the fact that the burdens of caregiving are a reality for families in resource-poor settings.

The purpose of organising initiatives such as the Home-Based Care Alliance is to shift the focus on care away from intellectual, professional-driven discussions about gender inequality, and towards empowerment strategies and organising; women who have taken up this burden may be able to find their own realistic solutions – whether it is fair compensation for their labour or to not perform the labour at all. Home-based caregivers who choose to do that important work in their communities should be supported to organise. Their status and role should also be formalised, for example through formal registration cards (as the Home-Based Care Alliance in Kenya is distributing). By formally recognising the people who choose to take on home-based care work and integrating them into formal healthcare systems, women in families would less often be left to deal informally with HIV/AIDS.

A distinction must be drawn between women who have taken on home-based care for the community, and those who are forced to take on the burden of care for family members. This chapter refers primarily to women (and men) who are providing home-based care services for the community (not just their immediate family members) and who are organised into groups. There have been increased calls for salaries or stipends for caregivers to remunerate there efforts. The founders of the Home-Based Care Alliance envisioned a federation of caregiver groups who could make their work sustainable through collective enterprise. An empowerment focus suggests that only solutions emanating from caregivers themselves, through process and dialogues led by organised groups of home-based caregivers will prove themselves truly sustainable. This case study aims to prove that grassroots women are both ideally placed to improve governance processes related to AIDS and development, and therefore entitled to greater representation in decision-making due to their singular and vital contributions to mitigating HIV/AIDS.

Case Study: The Kakamega District Home-Based Care Alliance: A Grassroots Women's Initiative To Transform And Improve The Local Government's Response To AIDS

In Kenya, Grassroots Organizations Operating Together in Sisterhood (GROOTS) Kenya has been able to build a strong national network of women's self-help groups over the last 10 years. GROOTS Kenya was founded in 1995 as a response to the inadequate visibility of grassroots women in development programmes and those decision-making forums that directly affect them and their communities. GROOTS Kenya bridges this gap through initiatives that are community-centred and women-led. As a part of their organising, GROOTS Kenya has worked over the past year to found the

Home-Based Care Alliance. The idea to form an alliance of home-based caregivers emerged during the 2003 International Conference on AIDS and STIs in Africa, which was held in Nairobi, Kenya. There, home-based caregivers shared their work and experiences and asked donors to target more resources directly at the grassroots level. Representatives of the Global Fund in attendance claimed that there was no way for them to locate grassroots groups, which they characterized as marginal, small-scale and working in isolation (GROOTS Kenya, 2003). To counter these false stereotypes and raise the visibility of home-based caregivers' responses, GROOTS worked to facilitate home-based caregivers within its network to federate and organise themselves through mapping and consultation processes. Grassroots members of GROOTS Kenya launched the Kenyan Home-Based Care Alliance pilot in 2005.

The Kenyan Home-Based Care Alliance has built caregivers' capacities through peer learning and exchange, enhanced their livelihoods through sustainable collective enterprises (such as collective purchase of cows for milk sale, beekeeping and horticultural projects) and has served as a platform for negotiating with stakeholders and decision-makers for key resources within the community through ongoing consultations and special meetings called local-to-local dialogues. In these ways, the Alliance has added value to the ongoing work of caregivers as they provide essential services to the communities in which members live and work – enabling the sick to access care and support and legal resources for cases of asset stripping and disinheritance, as well as providing a platform for marginalised groups, who often feel the worst effects of the epidemic, to be heard and take action through participation in support groups and becoming caregivers themselves. In addition to providing essential support to vulnerable community members affected by the epidemic, the Alliance has united caregivers and draws recognition to grassroots work. The Alliance has increased home-based caregivers' confidence and capacity through peer learning exchanges on caregiving skills, organising and negotiation methodologies such as the local-to-local dialogue to represent their work and participate in the decision-making processes that will be described below. As the self-help groups are linked in a national network with ongoing dialogue and consultation, they are able to share and analyse their strategies

The Shibuye Community Health Workers, who have worked since 1999 to support and care for HIV-positive community members, led the process of federating caregiving groups to form the Home-Based Care Alliance in Kenya's Western Province.[4] Shibuye began organising the Alliance through an action research mapping process in which members first collected and compiled data on caregiving groups that they already knew about. They then led a more rigorous process of locating, forming relationships with and collecting the same information on previously unknown groups. Through the mapping process, grassroots leaders mobilised 17 new groups (1,812 caregivers) to join the Alliance and found out that by federating the group, they collectively cared for 2,276 people living with HIV and AIDS, 6,000 orphans, 2,000 widows and 4,000 other needy people (GROOTS Kenya 2006). The mapping process enabled Shibuye to clearly articulate to local authorities and other stakeholders the contributions they were making and the positive impact they were having on the community.

The group began as a team of health workers caring for HIV-positive members of the community, and has grown into a strong network that has developed partnerships with local leadership and significantly influenced decision-making structures to increase the support for HIV-positive community members, as well as gained recognition for their work as a constituency. Shibuye has been leading this process as founding members of the Kakamega District Home-Based Care Alliance. The district Alliance is an example of a grassroots effort that has provided extensive support to HIV-positive community members, including direct care, increased access to medicines and referral services. Beyond these more obvious caregiving tasks, the Alliance has helped to open up space for those directly affected by HIV/AIDS to voice their needs and concerns to those who make decisions on policies and resources related to HIV/AIDS.

As the needs of those living with HIV have changed over time, due in part to greater access to ART and other medications, increased access to information and improved palliative care, caregivers' roles have changed. When GROOTS Kenya began its home-based care work in 1999, caregivers primarily provided direct care to bedridden patients. Their work has now expanded to include a range of tasks such as providing assistance in administering and managing medications, ensuring treatment adherence, supporting orphans and linking to medical, financial and livelihood resources available within the community for those affected by the pandemic (Huairou Commission 2007). For example, as women and children have become widowed or orphaned, caregivers have taken a lead in supporting affected community members to secure land entitlements and other assets that are often lost when husbands and fathers die. Caregivers have also raised community awareness to address stigma and discrimination and to reverse isolation, which has led to the development of a positive women-led support network within the Alliance.

Using the data gathered during the mapping process, leaders of the Shibuye Community Health Workers began engaging local leaders both formally and informally. Informally, they regularly arranged face-to-face meetings with local chiefs and CACC officers, in which they shared information on widow and orphan disinheritance, domestic violence and how their group was caring for such marginalised community members who were generally outside the reach of public services. The Shibuye Community Health Workers also conducted local-to-local dialogues in partnership with GROOTS Kenya on behalf of the Alliance, in which they arranged public dialogue sessions between grassroots caregivers and local leaders to share caregivers' perspectives, discuss challenges within the community and develop collaborative solutions.[5]

The group began by calling the CACC officers and informing them of their plan to support and reinforce what the government was doing, and letting them know that they were not attempting to criticise or point out CACC failures. For the community, the CACC was an entity that was difficult to access and not transparent. The solution was to mobilise all the community stakeholders to come together in a dialogue session. The group approached the provincial administrators who have power in the community but are also held accountable if they do not respond to the calls by the community. They also approached their local chief and asked the district officer to participate in the meetings. The chief and the district officer are both accessible to the community as they are located within it and were therefore already familiar with the work of the Alliance (Shivutse 2007).

Prior to the local-to-local dialogue, the Alliance consulted with the community in order to raise some of the priority issues to discuss with the stakeholders. These issues included lack of transparency as to who receives CACC funding, lack of sustainability of the projects and programmes that received CACC funding (short-term feeding programs, blanket distribution to orphans, etc.), and ensuring that the funds go to those people who are experienced in home-based care. In addition, many community members were concerned that those who are reviewing proposals within the CACC are political actors who may not be aware of who is active and experienced in the community, and were therefore giving funding to groups outside the community in other constituencies. It was important from the community perspective to provide information to the CACC on who the groups are that are working in the area (ibid.)

After the meeting, the community stakeholders agreed to track the resources available, identify existing groups in the area and look at the structures that are in place to coordinate with the CACC. The community also demonstrated that they were knowledgeable of the NACC strategic plan through which the CACCs all operate. They had been made aware of this information through membership in the national and international networks of GROOTS Kenya and GROOTS International, both of which have facilitated grassroots women's participation in policy and networking venues such as the International Conference on AIDS and STIs in Africa and the International AIDS Conference, among others (GROOTS Kenya 2003; Huairou Commission 2007)

By demonstrating that the Alliance members were making clear contributions and were aware of the priorities of the government, the decision-making structure recognised the group as integral to the process of distributing information about when the CACC is funding, what their priority areas would be, and who/what groups were being funded to work in those areas. The relationship is now collaborative instead of operating autonomously without knowledge of what the other was doing. Through Shibuye's leadership, the Kakamega District Home-Based Care Alliance now has official partnership status with the Shinyalu division CACC Officer. The Alliance provides an eye into the community, collecting data, statistics and information on vulnerabilities, as well as tracking and overseeing indigenous responses organised by caregivers.

As a result of the dialogue and ongoing engagement, the Alliance has also developed a formal partnership with the Kakamega District Office. This partnership designates the Alliance as official 'community responders' and provides them with office space, occasional funds for local projects, and the use of a vehicle to reach distant cases. The relationship also gives the group authority to intervene on women's and children's issues, such as domestic violence and land/property grabbing in collaboration with the provincial administration. The caregivers' role in this relationship is important in realising women's rights as they bridge the gap between the administration and citizens. On the one hand, district officers are generally male, and often from a different region and tribe. This means that they may not understand the local culture dictating relationships between women and men, and that women and children will probably not feel comfortable approaching them on issues as sensitive as domestic violence. On the other hand, women and children very often do not know or understand their rights or the administrative officials that are responsible for their enforcement. So the caregivers raise awareness of those rights and the institutions and systems in place for redressing grievances, and bring cases of violations from the victims to the administration (Shivutse 2008)

The Kakamega District Officer in particular sees this as a strategic partnership enabling his officers, mainly chiefs and sub-chiefs, to work hand-in-hand with local communities in addressing community problems (Romo 2007). The partnership has both simplified and supported his work. The District Officer also holds the authority to enforce the law in preventing land grabbing, denial of care and violence, and recognises that by backing Alliance members with such authority he can both better serve his constituency and validate Alliance members' interventions. For the Alliance, this partnership ensures that they have a voice within the District decision-making structures, and enables them to access resources and provides a route for community members who depend on the caregivers to seek recourse for violations of their rights. As a result of their work, several cases of land grabbing and illegal land sales have been prevented, and several cases of child and wife abuse have been redressed.

The Kakamega District Home-Based Care Alliance has directly and successfully dealt with many of the challenges of decentralisation laid out in the previous discussion. The shifts are summarised in the table below. As the table makes clear, caregivers have been able to fill the gap between the existing administrative structures and the communities, thereby increasing transparency, accountability and disseminating information between communities and officials.

Members of Kakamega Home-Based Care Alliance have demonstrated the capacity of grassroots women to effectively respond to local needs and

Table 4.1 What has shifted due to grassroots women' organizing and partnership-building in Kakamega

Prior to Dialogue	*Since Dialogue*
Lack of funding transparency	Communities know where CACC funding is going
Unsustainable and briefcase NGOs being supported by CACC	Sustainable, local organizations identified by the community, including quality home-based care groups receiving support
CACC and District Officers didn't have information about how many people had AIDS	Accurate statistics being collected and shared by home-based caregivers
Government and community groups working in isolation from each other	Community groups and government working in collaboration

provide a platform for those most affected by AIDS to voice their needs and concerns from their own perspectives. Grassroots women taking leadership in forming the Kakamega District Home-Based Care Alliance initiated the process without outside resources. Their aim was to meet the unmet needs of the sick, abandoned and dispossessed, through both directly supporting them and also bringing the attention of the general public and local authorities to their contributions. By partnering with CACC and the District Office, they set a precedent for a new way to forge partnerships between civil society and local authorities to improve the AIDS response. Through the organisation and intervention of the Alliance in Kakamega, an increasing amount of public funds now directly reach those that the community itself identifies as being in need, rather than being diverted to a select few and/or being mismanaged by unscrupulous officials. Caregivers are continuing to educate local authorities on community needs and means of improving the effectiveness of their programs. In addition to forming direct links between the community and the local administration, caregivers are also at the forefront of bringing recognition to grassroots women as key stakeholders in AIDS responses. Rather than acting as victims of the pandemic or beneficiaries in the response, the grassroots women leaders of the Kakamega Alliance has shown that women can be active participants in improving governance and local responses to HIV/AIDS, to ensure that they work for women and communities.

Conclusion

This case study has demonstrated the ways that organised groups of home-based caregivers are holding the institutions that are supposed to serve them and their communities to account. In conclusion, we recommend a number of actions that various stakeholders in the global AIDS response can take to support such community-driven actions and to replicate these results so that the potential of communities – who play a vital part in the national AIDS response – is fully utilised, and to ensure that the AIDS response, to which billions of dollars have been committed, is governed well from the perspective of those who are bearing the heaviest burden of the pandemic. This case study and the lessons to be learned from it have far-reaching policy implications for multilateral and bilateral donors, academics and policy-making institutions. The experiences of the Kakamega District Home-Based Care Alliance illustrate the opportunities presented by the establishment to decentralised funding structures, and the factors necessary for grassroots constituencies to take advantage of those opportunities. The Home-Based Care Alliance in Kakamega shows how local responses to AIDS, including decentralised funding mechanisms, can operate successfully.

Grassroots women are actors for strong governance and their communities in the context of AIDS, and their initiatives should be acknowledged, resourced and built upon. As they respond to HIV and AIDS, and attempt to improve the quality of care for their community, women are improving governance processes by bringing vital information about the community to decision-makers via consultations, dialogues, advice and direct participation in government processes. They identify priorities, articulate what is not functioning and propose collaborative solutions. As constituency-based organisations with wide-ranging and diverse networks, grassroots women's groups ensure that the priorities of those most affected by HIV are represented on CACCs and community development funds, and that the resources from them are getting to those in the community who are most in need. In this way, grassroots women in partnership with local authorities are effectively countering resource capture by local elites and through nepotism, and promoting transparency and community accountability.

Members of the Home-Based Care Alliance in Kakamega, armed with their first-hand knowledge of the community, were able to express the needs and challenges of the community to CACC and district officers, make recommendations for channelling funding to sustainable organisations, thereby building the capacity of the local government to fulfil the responsibilities placed on it by increasingly decentralised structures. It is therefore clear that organising processes led by grassroots women – whether they are rural women, slum dwellers, people living with HIV/AIDS (PLWHAs), or others – must be supported. Organising needs to be pre-resourced and core funding for organising needs to be sustainable. Organising and networking at the national and international level also needs to be supported to enable information-sharing and peer learning. Private donors know this and have been supporting organising processes for years. But the level at which they are able to fund is inadequate to get these organising processes to scale. Large donors – bilateral and multilateral – need to commit their resources to organising processes in an ongoing way.

It is widely recognised that decentralisation does not *a priori* create more accountable or democratic funding or decision-making at the local level. Large public funds are an opportunity for fostering public accountability and good governance via the grassroots constituencies that are most affected by decision-making. Yet without ensuring that funding and decision-making structures include participatory consultative mechanisms to include community voices in their processes, local authorities often tend to reinforce power structures. Furthermore, local authorities and other government officials, particularly in resource-poor settings, do not always have the capacity or resources to coordinate effective responses on their own. In Kakamega, this led to CACC funding being channelled to unsustainable AIDS programs and briefcase NGOs. Grassroots women in Kakamega and elsewhere have been able to effectively counter these challenges through their organisational and partnership-building activities. Using their standing in the community and the trust they gained through their ongoing work as home-based caregivers, the Shibuye Home-Based Caregivers were able to facilitate a local-to-local dialogue process with the community, where they were able to identify issues and priorities, and dialogue with local government officials to create concrete solutions. Since the community clearly trusted the caregivers, local government began to depend on them as their 'eye to the community.' With trusted caregivers sitting in the district office and serving as advisors to CACC, the community correspondingly begins to place more trust in the government.

National governments and institutions such as UNAIDS and the World Bank, which have assisted national governments to create national AIDS councils, and donors that are currently funding them, have a responsibility to ensure effective operation of community-level AIDS councils and distribution of funding at the community level. If funding is supposed to be reaching the community level, quotas for the percentage of money guaranteed to reach that level should be declared. Furthermore, representatives of organised constituencies need to be involved in decision-making bodies such as CACCs and NACCs to counter token representation of groups such as women, CSOs and people living with AIDS.

A holistic, multisectoral response to HIV/AIDS, which addresses governance at every level, is needed in order to create an effective national AIDS response. The Kakamega District Home-Based Care Alliance showcases one type of initiative at the community level, and the transformation of the AIDS response in that community provides a justification for including community-based organisations, particularly those composed of home-based caregivers, as actors on an equal footing with other stakeholders in community, national and global AIDS responses.

Notes

1 With Esther Mwaura-Muiru, Violet Shivutse and Anna Williams. This chapter was written prior to the presidential elections in late 2007. Special thanks to the following people for vastly improving this paper at every step along its long route to completion: Michael Cohen, Jan Peterson, Sarah Silliman, Sandra Schilen, Esther Mwaura-Muiru, Everlyne Nairesiae, Stephen Lewis, Blerta Cela and Sophie Harman.

2 For a comprehensive overview of National AIDS Authorities' roles and functions, see: Clare Dickinson, *National AIDS Coordinating Authorities: A synthesis of lessons learned and taking learning forward*, DFID Health Resource Centre (London: 2005).
3 See World Bank Projects and Operations Database: http://web.worldbank.org/WBSITE/EXTERNAL/PROJECTS/0,menuPK:41389~pagePK:95863~piPK:95983~tgDetMenuPK:228424~tgProjDetPK:73230~tgProjResPK:95917~tgResMenuPK:224076~theSitePK:40941,00.html and Global Fund Commitments and Disbursements Database: http://www.theglobalfund.org/en/funds_raised/commitments/
4 Shibuye is a location (an administrative unit similar to a town) within Shinyalu division of the Kakamega District.
5 Originally piloted in 2002 by six Huairou Commission members, including GROOTS Kenya, local-to-local dialogues are locally designed strategies whereby grassroots women's groups initiate and engage in ongoing dialogues with local authorities to negotiate a range of development issues and priorities to influence policies, plans and programs in ways that address women's priorities. Dialogues are convened by grassroots women and used to change the terms of negotiation between communities and their local authorities. For further information, read 'Local to Local Dialogue: A Grassroots Women's Perspective on Good Governance,' at http://www.huairou.org/knowledge/resource.html.

Bibliography

AIDS Campaign Team for Africa (ACTAfrica). (2006). *Implementing Multi-Country HIV/AIDS Programs (MAP) in Africa: Report on Africa Region HIV/AIDS Consultation in Civil Society Responses in MAP Projects* Washington DC: World Bank. May 2006.

Appadurai, Arjuan. (2001). 'Deep Democracy: Urban Governmentality and the Horizon of Politics' *Environment and Urbanization*, 13 (2), 23–43.

Barnett, T. and Whiteside, A. (1999). 'HIV/AIDS and Development: Case Studies and a Conceptual Framework' *European Journal of Development Research* 11(2): 220–34.

Brown, J.C., Ayvaliki, D. and Mohammad, N. (2004). *Turning Bureaucrats into Warriors: Preparing and Implementing Multi-Sector HIV/AIDS in Africa, A General Operations Manual.* Washington, DC: The International Bank for Reconstruction and Development/The World Bank.

Caldwell, J.C. (2000). 'Rethinking the African AIDS Epidemic' *Population and Development Review.* 26(1): 117–35.

Campbell, T. (2003). *The Quiet Revolution: Decentralisation and the Rise of Political Participation in Latin American Cities.* Pittsburgh, PA: The University of Pittsburgh Press.

De Waal, A. (1997). 'Democratizing the aid encounter in Africa' *International Affairs* 73(4).

Dickinson, C. (2005). *National AIDS Coordinating Authorities: A synthesis of lessons learned and taking learning forward.* DFID Health Resource Centre. London: Department for International Development.

Earthtrends Website Searchable Database. World Resources Institute (2003). http://www.earthtrends.wri.org

Gordon, G. (1995). 'Participation, Empowerment and Sexual Health in Africa' in Gary Craig and Marjorie Mayo (Eds) *Community Empowerment: A Reader in Participation and Development* London: Zed Books.

GROOTS Kenya. (2003). '13th ICASA Community Caucus Report'.

—— (2006). 'Home-Based Care Alliance Mapping Report'.

Hadiz, V.R. (2003). 'Decentralisation and Democracy in Indonesia: A Critique of Neo-Institutionalist Perspectives' *Southeast Asia Research Centre Working Paper Series* No. 47.

Helling, L., Serrano, R. and Warren, D. (2005). 'Linking Community Empowerment, Decentralised Governance, and Public Service Provision Through a Local Development Framework' *Social Protection Discussion Paper* No. 0535. Washington, DC: The World Bank.

Huairou Commission. (2005). *Kenya AIDS Watch.* February (Available at http://huairou.org/assets/download/Watch_report_AIDS.pdf).

—— (2007). *Uniting Communities Around Caregiving: Grassroots Women's Perspectives on the HIV and AIDS Pandemic. A Report from the Grassroots Women's International Academy and YWCA International Women's Summit.*

Hunt, C.W. (1989). 'Migrant Labor and Sexually Transmitted Disease: AIDS in Africa' *Journal of Health and Social Behavior* 30(4).

Joint UN Programme on HIV/AIDS (UNAIDS)/World Health Organization (2004). *AIDS Epidemic Update.* Geneva: UNAIDS.

Joint UN Programme on HIV/AIDS (UNAIDS). (2004). *Kenya: National AIDS Control Council Joint Institutional Review* Nairobi: UNAIDS.

Kenya National AIDS Control Council. (2000). *Kenya National HIV and AIDS Strategic Plan.* Nairobi: NACC.

Mehta, A.K and Gupta, S. (2006). *The Impact of HIV/AIDS on Women Caregivers in Situations of Poverty: Policy Issues.* The United Nations Development Fund for Women.

National Research Council of the National Academies. (2003). *Cities Transformed: Demographic Change and Its Implications in the Developing World.* Washington, DC: National Academies Press.

Olenja, J. (1999). 'Assessing Community Attitudes towards Home-Based Care for People with AIDS (PWAs) in Kenya' *Journal of Community Health* 24(3).

Oyaya, C.O. and Rifkin, S.B. (2003). 'Health Sector reforms in Kenya: an examination of district level planning' *Health Policy,* 64:113–27.

Poku, N.K. (2002). 'Poverty, Debt and Africa's HIV/AIDS Crisis' *International Affairs* 78(3)531–46.

Razavi, S. (2007). *The Political and Social Economy of Care in a Development Context: Contextual Issues, Research Questions and Policy Options.* United Nations Research Institute for Social Development, Gender and Development Paper Number 3.

Republic of Kenya. (2006). *United Nations Special Session on HIV/AIDS 2006 Country Report.*

Romo, J.M. (January 2007). Interview.

Shivutse, V. (January 2007). Interview.

—— (2008). Interview.

Strickland, R. (2004). *To Have and to Hold: Women's Property and Inheritance Rights in the Context of HIV/AIDS in Sub-Saharan Africa.* Washington, DC: International Center for Research on Women.

Ström, M-Louise. (2005). *Citizens at the Centre: AIDS Councils as Catalysts for Unlocking Citizen Power.* Pretoria, South Africa: The Institute for Democracy in South Africa.

United Nations. (2001). 'On the Socio-economic Impact of HIV/AIDS' *Population and Development Review* 27(3): 619–24.

Urdang, S. (2006). 'The Care economy: Gender and the silent AIDS crisis in Southern Africa' *Journal of Southern African Studies* 32(1): 165–77.

Whiteside, A. (2002). 'Poverty and HIV/AIDS in Africa' *Third World Quarterly* 23 (2):313–32.

World Bank Project Document No. PID9280. (2000). *Kenya AIDS Disaster Response Project* Project ID KEPE70920. 2000.

World Health Organization. (2007). *Report on the Eastern and Southern Africa Regional Meeting on Nutrition and HIV/AIDS.*

Part III

Partnerships: public-private, formal and informal networks

5 Business and the governance of HIV/AIDS in South Africa

Antoinette Handley[1]

In addition to planting the seed of manifold human tragedies, South Africa's HIV/AIDS epidemic – one of the most serious anywhere – is challenging the roles and function of the country's core economic and political actors. Conventionally, for example, we would expect the government to spearhead the national response to the pandemic, yet the South African government has been curiously remiss in this regard. Conversely, in 2002 the South African mining company Anglo American (which over the years has been the target of much criticism for its labour practices) announced that *it* would provide antiretroviral (ARV) drugs to its employees. It seems a strange reversal of roles, for business to take on health and welfare functions that are conventionally expected of the state, inviting speculation that this might presage a 'change in the meaning of government' in South Africa (Rhodes 1996: 652). There is much here that is congruent with Rhodes' definition of governance, as self-organizing inter-organisational networks – in this case, companies – which have reacted in a variety of ways to government's conspicuous failure on this issue. These networks are, Rhodes tells us, a 'pervasive feature' of service delivery in societies where the state has hollowed out. While the government's stance on the epidemic has attracted much attention – as has civil society's mobilisation around this issue – less academic attention has been paid to the varied reactions of the country's business community. This paper seeks to address that gap, focusing on the role of the private sector in the governance of HIV/AIDS-affected South Africa, and the issues and problems arising from this.

This chapter explores a number of interrelated sets of questions. First, how has the South African private sector responded to the country's epidemic? Here it is important to disaggregate 'business' as a category, as responses have varied widely within the sector, across time, across firm size and across sectors of the economy. Second, how can we account for these variations? The chapter concludes by considering the capacity of business to respond effectively to the epidemic and the limitations of both public and private sector-based responses. The reader should be warned that what follows is based on only preliminary research. Definitive conclusions concerning the various hypotheses await further carefully structured comparative fieldwork.

Governance of HIV/AIDS in South Africa

When we consider who should respond at the domestic level to the HIV/AIDS crisis, most often we think first of national governments.[2] Yet across Sub-Saharan Africa, the reality is that many governments lack both real incentives and the institutional capacity to act with the requisite urgency and scale (De Waal 2006; Patterson 2005). Even for those states that have both the will and the means to respond, the measures that are necessary may run counter to the last 25 years of neo-liberal policy prescriptions, which have disempowered the state and curtailed its reach (Poku and Whiteside 2004).[3]

The private sector is less often considered an important respondent to the crisis, yet it may have both the means and the motivation to react – after all, HIV/AIDS is impacting not only the health of African populations, but also their economies. Faced with the prospect of economic slowdown, declining profits and challenges to its ability to procure labour and sustain a customer base, business has an urgent set of incentives that galvanise its response to the crisis.[4] Moreover, in the short and medium term, the many decisions taken by thousands of firms will directly impact the lives of hundreds of thousands of employees. Over the long term, millions will likely be affected by the capacity of business, working in concert with or in opposition to government, to respond to the crisis in ways that might bolster the future resilience of the political economy. It is important, therefore, to map these developments and consider their implications for the capacity of South African society to respond adequately to the epidemic.

Background

With respect to HIV/AIDS at least, South Africa presents a dramatic crisis of governance, namely the failure of the state to itself respond adequately to the epidemic, let alone to cooperate with other social actors in their attempts to do so. It was not obvious ahead of time that this would be the case; on the contrary, many had hoped to see much more effective governance on HIV/AIDS as the country democratized in the mid 1990s. Following decades of white minority rule under apartheid, African National Congress (ANC), led by Nelson Mandela, swept to power in South Africa's first democratic elections in 1994. They carried with them the hopes of millions of South Africans that this electoral triumph would usher in a new kind of governance: one that better served their needs and would respond with careful and sustained compassion to the development challenges that shaped their everyday lives. In the 13 years since then, the democratically elected government (now under the leadership of Thabo Mbeki) made significant progress, extending basic services (including the free provision of healthcare to pregnant women and to children under the age of five, and the expansion of access to low-income housing and to electricity) to a large swathe of previously underserved citizens (Handley 2004; Policy Coordination and Advisory Services 2004).

Many of these successes, however, have been overshadowed by failure in a critical policy area: by all accounts, the South African government has failed dismally to respond to the country's devastating HIV/AIDS epidemic.[5] The South African epidemic, it must be said, is one of the world's most acute: there are currently 5.5 million South Africans living with HIV, a prevalence of 18.8 per cent among adults aged 15–49 years, and some 1.2 million AIDS orphans (UNAIDS 2006). A number of interrelated factors have significantly hindered the capacity of the country's public sector to react consistently and constructively to the growing crisis. There is no room to discuss these in any detail here, but these factors include the curious stance adopted by President Mbeki in highlighting 'denialist' views on the connection between HIV and AIDS; the ongoing racialisation of the epidemic and of responses to it; and the way in which the issue became part of a fiercely contested and partisan pattern of politics in South Africa.[6]

Given this background, what are the prospects that South African business can contribute to a broadly based governance response to HIV/AIDS? There is no question that the South African economy supports one of the largest, most powerful and most diverse – in terms at least of sub-sectors of the economy – private sectors in Africa. If there is any African business community that has the institutional and financial capacity to mount a concerted response to the epidemic, it is this one. Moreover, it is arguable that the gap left by government's failure provides South African business with an especially compelling set of incentives to respond constructively.

Some background about the South African private sector may be in order here. The country's agricultural settler economy was transformed, first by the discovery of gold and diamonds in the late 1800s, and then by a process of industrialisation and strong economic growth up through the 1960s. Consequently, by the late twentieth century, the South African economy was highly diversified producing a range of manufactured goods and serviced by a sophisticated financial sector. In 2000, manufacturing and industry contributed 44 per cent of gross domestic product (GDP), and services comprised 51 per cent (World Bank 2000). However, while the economy was growing increasingly diversified, the ownership and management of that economy remained overwhelmingly in white hands. Not only was it extraordinarily difficult for black South Africans to create or operate businesses, but ownership too was restricted to the small white community. For much of the twentieth century, the South African economy was notoriously oligopolistic, and it remains so in some important sectors. English-speakers dominated South African business for most of the country's colonial history and, following the discovery of the country's mineral wealth, a few large firms came to own an extraordinarily large share of the country's stock exchange [in the mid 1990s, just five business groups controlled more than 70 per cent of the assets listed on the Johannesburg Stock Exchange (JSE)] (McGregor 2004). This boosted the political and economic influence of these firms in the political economy.

In accord with the received wisdom of the day, South African industrial policy from the 1950s to the 1970s included a strong element of protectionism, exercised principally via the use of tariffs and subsidies. This relative lack of competitiveness was exacerbated with the political turbulence of 1970s and 1980s as financial and trading sanctions (and consequent foreign exchange regulations) restricted both external investment into South Africa by foreigners, and limited international investment opportunities for large South African firms outside of the country. Instead, already substantial and market-dominant South African firms were forced to expand their buyouts of shares of other South African firms, further increasing their economic dominance. This isolation from international markets and the marked degree of domestic oligopoly inevitably produced distortions and inefficiencies within the market over time. Then, over the course of the 1990s, the ANC government introduced a significant shift in direction, adopting a surprisingly conservative set of macroeconomic policies which significantly liberalised the country's trade.[7] These measures had a profound effect on South African business, forcing many firms to restructure themselves in order to become more globally competitive – and also provided the challenging context in which business would be forced to respond to the AIDS epidemic.[8]

As a country with a long-standing and relatively powerful private sector, South Africa has long developed a large number of business organisations to represent diverse business interests, ranging from small sector-specific lobbies to large, economy-wide federations. These organisations were, mostly long-standing, well-resourced and well-institutionalised, at least in comparison with those found in other African economies. Furthermore, in the late 1990s, a new business association – the South African Business Coalition on HIV/AIDS (SABCOHA) – was formed specifically to coordinate and encourage private sector responses to the epidemic. This predated similar developments at the international level, such as the Global Business Coalition on HIV/AIDS, Tuberculosis and Malaria (GBC) that was formed in 2001 to coordinate the efforts of multinational firms on similar issues.[9]

Business and HIV/AIDS

In affected societies across the globe, businesses' responses to AIDS have been many and varied. Part of this variety may be attributed to the great diversity within the category of 'business' itself. After all, the collective term 'business' encapsulates a range of sizes of firms, from the smallest to the largest, engaged in a great variety of economic activities and located in different areas of the economy, comprising both national and multinational capital, and drawing on a range of diverse organisational styles and traditions.

The potential responses by firms may be equally various. Given the horror of the projected impact of the epidemic, firms may wish to transfer the costs of the epidemic to governments and private households, and many have indeed done so, not least by simply shedding large numbers of jobs.[10]

Nonetheless, a small number of firms have also responded with laudably comprehensive programmes for their employees. In South Africa, legislation does not legally require firms to respond constructively to the epidemic;[11] this means that HIV/AIDS interventions by the private sector are not regarded as a legal requirement but must be seen either as a voluntarily assumed corporate social responsibility (CSR; Root 2007), or as a prudent, business-minded response to a strategic threat in the overall economic environment. Beyond a schematic sense of the broad range of responses, we know surprisingly little about how firms are responding – and why specific firms respond in specific ways.

In considering the range of potential outcomes, it is possible to characterise firm responses as more or less constructive. For the purposes of this chapter, by a constructive response I mean specifically one that is likely to advance and contribute to broader society-wide attempts to mitigate the effects and spread of the epidemic. This kind of response from a firm stands in contrast, therefore, with those firms who simply do nothing or who actively seek to transfer the costs of the epidemic to other actors. In what follows, this chapter will draw on an existing political economy literature, developed mostly to account for firms' behaviour with respect to economic policy, to develop some hypotheses concerning how best to account for firm responses to the HIV/AIDS epidemic.

Why – and how – South African business has responded to the epidemic

In the absence of conclusive evidence and on the basis of as yet only preliminary research then, we may nonetheless hypothesise that certain kinds of firms are more likely to respond constructively to the AIDS epidemic than others. While the political science literature on business in the developing world does not directly address the HIV/AIDS epidemic, we can extrapolate compelling (and oftentimes competing) sets of explanations for how firms are likely to respond to a crisis such as this from two of the discipline's established intellectual traditions. The first set of explanations, rooted in political economy and rational-actor approaches to firm behaviour, focuses on the variable economic impact of the epidemic and predicts that those firms whose profitability are most severely affected by the epidemic are most likely to respond to that epidemic.[12] The second set of explanations focuses on the pressures emanating from the 'moral economy'; various strands within this tradition argue that firms' responsiveness will be driven by broader political and institutional factors, including governments' own level of responsiveness, the levels of public pressure on the issue, the political identity of those most adversely affected by the epidemic, and the institutional history and established practices of the firms concerned.

The first of these arguments focuses on the *economic/structural* variables that shape the responses of business, namely how the epidemic affects the firm's bottom line (Drummond and Kelly 2006; Friedman 1970). The impact of the HIV/AIDS epidemic across any given population may vary dramatically by race, class, gender, occupation, and/or education levels (Barnett and Whiteside 2002; Epstein 2007). This means that the epidemic will necessarily affect every economy – and the specific profitability of a particular firm in a specific economic sub-sector – slightly differently. Different sub-sectors have different labour requirements, in terms of both the numbers of people employed and their skills levels. The epidemic also affects their different customer bases and marketing strategies. Different sub-sectors also have distinct time horizons within which they need to recoup their investments. A framework that considers the dynamics of the particular political economy of each firm also needs to control for the sub-sector of the economy in which a firm operates.

By contrast, the moral economy framework directs our attention to a second set of factors – *political/social* factors. This group of approaches draws attention to the role of historical patterns and the development of social and economic institutions. It specifically identifies the significance of the politics of the particular society with which we are concerned. Governments, for example, provide the context and the rules that shape the environment within which business acts. Even in situations of 'embedded autonomy,' states generate the milieu within which firms operate. An organised, predictable public sector response to the epidemic arguably will allow business in turn to effectively confront risk and generate long-sighted responses (Evans 1995). From this vantage point, a high level of responsiveness by the state facilitates a similarly responsive set of strategies by the private sector (Maxfield and Schneider 1997). The economic/structural view, by contrast, would suggest the opposite; in terms of this logic, if government was already responding to the problem, a 'rational' economic actor would prefer to do nothing, i.e. to 'free-ride'.

Even though no such metrics are available for civil society, it is important to consider also what the non-state sources of pressure on business are (Vogel 2005), and how they may prompt firms to respond.[13] These pressures can be expressed by extensive media coverage, mobilised popular sentiment and the activities of pressure groups (Bor 2007).[14] Demographic factors are also potentially important. Given the scale of HIV/AIDS in South Africa, the epidemic clearly impacts the country's national demographics (for example by disproportionately affecting women and the 15–40 age group). This in turn shapes the *economic* impact of the epidemic, and hence could potentially shape the political responses of individual firms. It is therefore important to consider the extent to which factors such as race, gender and class create political pressures for business to act. Gauri and Lieberman argue that boundaries set up by pre-existing political identities shape governments' responsiveness (Gauri and Lieberman 2006). The same dynamics might apply to firms.

Historical institutionalists argue that existing pathways incline actors toward particular responses.[15] This view predicts that where the private sector has historically demonstrated the organisational and institutional capacity to organise itself, either collectively or at a firm level, it is more likely to respond in a concerted fashion (Nabila *et al.* 2001; Schneider 2004). More specifically expressed, if certain sub-sectors have a strong tradition of CSR, or if particular firms have historically assumed a relatively expansive set of health and welfare responsibilities for their workers, this will arguably generate a more constructive response to the epidemic.

Based on these broad hypotheses, we can speculate that firm responsiveness in South Africa will be shaped by the following five factors:

i. Firm capacity: Large, well established firms with the financial and human resources to focus on this issue are more likely to respond than small, informal firms with limited operating budgets and planning horizons;
ii. Firm profitability: Firms whose profitability are most drastically affected are most likely to respond (This is particularly true of those firms whose profitability is affected because of their labour profile. As yet, few firms appear to be fundamentally restructuring their business or even their business strategies because of an anticipated impact on their customers. Some of the large, discount retailers may be an exception here);
iii. A history of CSR: Firms who have a well-established institutional history of CSR and/or an expansive definition of their own responsibilities *vis-à-vis* their workers' health are more likely to respond constructively;
iv. Political pressure: Firms who are targeted by high profile media and public attention, non-governmental organisation (NGO) activism and/or union campaigns are more likely to respond than those not so targeted; and
v. The broader political context: This factor could operate in one of two quite different ways. In a national context where government has not responded to the epidemic, business may feel obligated to step into the policy vacuum on the one hand. On the other hand, in a place like South Africa, the high levels of politicisation of the issue lying behind government's failure to act may equally serve to discourage business from reacting constructively, as it may hesitate to behave in a way seen to be critical of government or contrary to government's stance. Here we should consider too the role of race in shaping the course of the South African debate and policy-making.

In what follows, I consider these factors in more detail, examining how they play out in the actual decision-making of South African firms across selected sub-sectors of the economy.

The capacity of individual firms to tackle the crisis

Both Uganda and South Africa are experiencing severe, high-profile and regionalised HIV/AIDS epidemics. In South Africa, however, the private sector appears to have responded to that epidemic in a much more concerted, proactive and high-profile way (at least certain firms have) than is commonly visible in Uganda.[16] On the face of it, our first hypothesis – concerning firm capacity – provides a clear and striking explanation for these different national levels of responsiveness by the private sector. As outlined above, the South African private sector is Africa's largest, most diverse and structurally most powerful. In Uganda by contrast, the country's private sector is smaller, even as a proportion of the smaller Ugandan economy. Ugandan firms themselves are also, for the most part, smaller than their South African counterparts, and Ugandan businesses generally employ fewer people and wield smaller budgets. Firms in Uganda thus have little political, financial or institutional capacity to tackle the epidemic on their own. Strikingly, the same relationship between firm size/capacity and responsiveness is repeated *within* South Africa, where it is for the most part, large, well-established firms that have responded constructively, while smaller businesses have demonstrated little capacity to develop holistic or proactive responses.[17]

From this perspective then, it seems obvious why business in South Africa responded more effectively than in Uganda; it is simply much larger, better institutionalised and has greater financial resources. The problem with this argument, however, is that in terms of this logic, one would expect similar dynamics from the respective public sectors of these two countries. That is, one would expect that the South African state, which is significantly larger and better resourced than the Ugandan state, would be more likely to respond constructively to the epidemic. Yet, as we know, the South African government has failed to respond while the Ugandan government has led a response to the epidemic that is widely regarded as one of the world's most impressive (Allen and Heald 2004; Putzel 2004). Moreover, even staying within the realm of the private sector, not all large firms (be they South African or Ugandan) have responded constructively. Resources and capacity, therefore, may be a necessary but not a sufficient condition for a constructive response.

The macroeconomics of HIV/AIDS in South Africa

In thinking about the connection between firm responsiveness and the impact of the epidemic on firm profitability, what is perhaps most surprising is how little consensus there is among economists on the precise economic impact of the epidemic (Dixon *et al.* 2001): most agree that it will reduce growth, but it is not clear exactly how it will do so, or by how much. Nor is there agreement on how to model the shifting epidemiological dynamics as diverse populations and institutions respond in different and sometimes unexpected ways to the epidemic, thus shifting its trajectory.[18]

Despite the difficulties, the effort to try to map the macroeconomic impact of the epidemic is well underway in South Africa.[19] This may be explained by the prominence of the South African financial and insurance industries.[20] South Africa has a well-developed financial infrastructure, including a profitable home-grown insurance industry, which has, for at least a decade now, been developing detailed econometric projections of the likely impact of the crisis. While there is little direct evidence to this end, it seems reasonable to assume that these projections have influenced the responses of some South African firms and served as an 'early warning' of the looming crisis, even in the absence of injunctions from the state.[21] There was thus a sub-sector of the South Africa private sector that had a direct business incentive to warn both current and potential clients elsewhere in the private sector that they needed to think about – and plan for – the economic fallout of the epidemic (Fourie 2006). It is possible, therefore, that the diversity of firm responses in South Africa may be attributable to i) whether or not such projections have been developed and publicised; and, where such projections were developed, to ii) the diversity among the various prognoses concerning how the epidemic would impact the economy as a whole.

The relatively large number of econometric models and explicit scenario planning exercises in South Africa[22] make it possible for us to consider some of the messages that these models transmit to private sector decision-makers about how they ought to react. A number of these models suggest an economic impact that, to the layperson, might appear slighter – or at least less catastrophic – than one might at first imagine given the country's high prevalence levels. In an off-the-record discussion with me, one economist went so far as to suggest that, far from being an economic disaster, the epidemic might actually result in an increase in the overall level of GDP per capita in South Africa! In order to understand this view, one must first consider the particular demographics of the epidemic in South Africa.

South Africa's epidemic has, for some time, been felt most keenly in the ranks of the country's marginalised – and hence, among those least likely to impact significantly on the functioning of the formal economy. Those who are falling ill and dying have been mostly female,[23] and, until recently at least, were frequently unemployed and/or employed in the informal sector; they have been poor and hence have not been significant purchasers of goods and services in the economy. Moreover, they have been largely unskilled,[24] in an economy that suffers from a huge surplus of skilled labour – which means that they are easily replaced. From a moral standpoint, the stance and implications of this kind of analysis are horrifying.[25] But this view is being advanced in some quarters in all seriousness – and some business leaders may be implicitly counting on it.[26]

At any rate, it is clear that the particular demographic profile of the South African epidemic is economically and politically significant. First, the impact on the overall shape of the economy is likely to be profound. In particular, it may weight the current capital: labour ratio even further in favour of capital (Arndt and Lewis 2001). Since 1970, this ratio in South Africa has increased by 142 per cent![27] Employers might respond to the epidemic by speculating that it will make labour more expensive (via, for example, lower productivity, higher absenteeism, and higher drug and healthcare costs). In such a case, the epidemic may exacerbate the move to substitute capital for labour. This would be bad news for jobseekers in an economy that, even before the epidemic began to be felt, was not generating formal sector jobs at nearly the rate necessary to significantly affect overall levels of poverty and inequality. In the medium to long term, this trend might consequently undermine the political organisation of unskilled labour and boost the relative political power of business.[28]

Second, the demographics of the epidemic produce rather different outcomes for those firms that rely on unskilled labour as opposed to those that employ scarce, skilled labour. Labour-intensive industries are particularly susceptible to the epidemic – but even here, not all firms, and not all industries, have reacted the same way. It is therefore instructive to consider at some length the contrast between the mining and construction sub-sectors, both industries that depend heavily on unskilled labour. I will use this comparison to also consider the remaining hypotheses on our list.

Unskilled labour: Comparing mining and construction

As I argued at the beginning of this chapter, South African mining companies – some of them at least – have attracted significant press attention because of how early they began to develop a constructive set of responses to the epidemic, and how relatively far-reaching those responses were. In addition to workplace prevention programmes and fully funded workplace voluntary counselling and testing sites, for example, some firms have also provided access to ARVs for their staff (and in some instances for their immediate dependents too).[29] The costs of these programmes have not been nearly as high as was initially expected, both because of the steep decrease in drug costs, but also because the take-up rate of ARVs by HIV-positive miners has much lower than many expected. Nonetheless, it is significant that these firms were willing to commit themselves to funding what initially looked like fairly significant expenses on this score.

Along with mining, construction is one of the sub-sectors of the South African economy that has been directly and severely affected by the epidemic.[30] Like mining, construction shares a reliance on migrant labour and on unskilled labour; moreover, the formal construction industry maintains very close connections to the informal sector – precisely the categories of workers where prevalence is highest. Construction workers are also unlikely to enjoy access to private health insurance. Yet the responses by firms in this sector present a striking contrast with those in mining. Generally, the responses of construction firms have not been nearly as proactive as those of mining; instead, many construction firms have tended to simply fire sick workers.

There are a number of potential reasons for these divergent approaches. We could consider, for example, the different structure and profile of these two industries. The structure of the mining industry, it might be argued, has predisposed it to address more directly the predicament of sick miners, rather than simply to replace them. First, one may speculate about the importance of established labour organisations and of close team work in mining (not a feature of construction to the same extent): one sick worker, operating at lower levels of productivity, can impact on the overall productivity – and safety – of the larger team. The costs of one sick individual are thus magnified in the mining industry.[31] Moreover, the mining industry has a long history of unionisation and the National Union of Mineworkers (NUM) has actively engaged the Chamber of Mines on its approach to the epidemic, pressing the mines to adopt a progressive rather than punitive approach to miners infected with HIV.[32]

Second, mining is an industry that has a long and institutionalised history of assuming an expansive (albeit often intensely self-interested) set of responsibilities *vis-à-vis* its workers. I refer here to the long-standing establishment of mineworkers' compounds, including company provision of accommodation, canteens, beer halls and on-site clinics. Miserly as these facilities were in the earliest decades of mining, they have since improved as a result of outside scrutiny and the activism of workers unions, and created a historical precedent for these firms to think more expansively about how best to develop and maintain a productive workforce.

Third, the oligopolistic structure of the mining industry has granted industry leaders tremendous influence and the ability to establish a series of norms for other players in the sub-sector, and has also facilitated coordinated responses within the mining sub-sector.[33] Large mining houses have also been prominent in the development of CSR programmes more broadly, and have played a similar role with respect to setting the tone for the industry's CSR response to HIV/AIDS.[34]

Finally, the mining industry's costs in the South Africa economy are – literally and figuratively – sunk; they are therefore unavoidably long-term, and returns on those investments are bound up with the political and economic well-being of the country. It is this factor that no doubt prompted far-sighted leadership within the sub-sector, which was not always politically progressive, to nonetheless participate, along with others in a small group of business leaders, in pressing for the political reform of apartheid in the late 1980s. Similarly, it motivated the development of CSR programmes by the same firms; and it may be part of what is driving their response to the AIDS epidemic in the current era.

The construction industry looks rather different in terms of these same factors. Instead of being built around relatively cohesive, on-site work teams, the construction industry has increasingly turned to outsourcing and to the casualisation of its labour force.[35] More and more, the industry is able to provide only discontinuous employment for its shifting workforce. The labour structure of the construction industry thus facilitates the transfer of the costs of illness and morbidity either to individual households or to sub-contractors. Moreover, the absence of a rooted 'base' for worker activity (construction is, by definition, constantly on the move from site to site, unlike mining), means that construction has no history of providing for the social and health needs of its workers, beyond the occasional nod to workplace safety (Meintjes *et al.* 2007). Nor has the national structure of the construction industry fostered a concerted response. In contrast with the mining oligopolies, the construction sector is characterised by a much larger number of relatively small firms competing fiercely with each other. This effectively means that no one firm can act as an industry leader; neither is any single firm large enough to pressure other firms to adopt similar practices.

All of this has failed to foster any organised sub-sectoral leadership: in contrast with the highly organised Chamber of Mines, for example, the political leadership of the construction industry is fragmented and politically inexperienced. Exacerbating this in the South African context is the heavy reliance of the construction industry on government contracts – the state is undoubtedly the industry's single largest customer. Industry leaders in construction were further immobilised by the decidedly mixed signals coming from the executive on the need for a response to AIDS. Political sensitivity – a fear of being seen to be critical of government – and greater susceptibility to political pressure from government[36] may thus have reinforced an already strong tendency for the sub-sector to ignore the problem, and to allow the abundant supplies of unskilled labour to substitute for keeping existing workers healthy and productive. Meintjes *et al.* argue that the Construction Industry Development Board 'is political in nature and so is inevitably influenced by the South African political climate which has not engendered a culture of effective HIV/AIDS management' (Meintjes *et al.* 2007). The ambivalence within government circles thus gives this politically timid sub-sector of business (which is not keen to be seen to be on the 'wrong' side of a very hot political issue by government) a further excuse to simply do nothing.[37]

This comparison of the mining and construction industries appears to endorse the validity of at least two of our final three hypotheses. In particular, it seems clear that the profitability of South Africa's mining sector is unquestionably affected by high prevalence levels amongst its numerous employees. That mining has been at the forefront of constructive firm responses to the HIV/AIDS epidemic is not that surprising, but this economistic logic is confounded elsewhere. Consider the case of government (as an employer in this instance, not as a policy-maker): while there is mounting evidence of high levels of prevalence among the country's public sector nurses, teachers and police officers, and the costs of replacing these trained employees are extremely high (unlike the lower costs for replacing unskilled labour), government's response (again, as employer) suggests that political factors may trump economic considerations. Conversely, if one applies a similarly economistic rationale to sub-sectors that employ skilled employers, similar anomalies emerge. It is, for example, not surprising that IT firms in South Africa have done little to respond to the epidemic: while the industry is reliant on expensive and highly trained staff, few of these employees are HIV-positive. Yet, while similar dynamics pertain for the financial sub-sector, a number of firms here *have* invested significant resources in responding to HIV/AIDS.[38] Evidently, economic/structural factors account for much of the private sector response, but there are important anomalies that they cannot so readily explain. Our five hypotheses therefore provide an important framework from which to begin to consider the nature and motivation of firm responses, but it is evident that more careful comparative work is necessary to definitively adjudicate the significance of the various hypotheses.

The macropolitics of HIV/AIDS

Finally, I would like to specifically address the role of political pressure and the politics of race in driving – or retarding – firm responses. It is unquestionably important here to consider the institutional nature and history of individual firms, and how they have reacted to a broad set of political pressures – but we should consider too how business in aggregate has responded to the crisis. Here it is striking that, despite its relative size and power, organised business in South Africa has mostly been unable – or unwilling – to organise to lobby to transform government policy on this issue. By contrast, we can consider the relatively assertive campaign that business waged in the 1990s to shift the new ruling party, the ANC, away from its leftist orientation and to embrace conservative macroeconomic policy (Handley 2005). The fact that business leadership continues to be overwhelmingly white, alongside Mbeki's highly racialised perspective on the issue, has made business reluctant to push perhaps as strongly as it ought to have, and for government to address the crisis more effectively.[39] Instead, South African business has reacted in a fractured way with some firms devising relatively impressive in-house responses and others completely neglecting to do so, instead passing the horrendous costs of the epidemic onto individuals and private households. This political rectitude on the part of business speaks also to the broader political context: within a single national political context, the responses of South African firms have been greatly diverse. This suggests that within each of our country cases, divergent firm responses may depend more on the particular structure of the firm and industry – but only a more systematic comparison of equivalent firms in other countries could determine this for sure.

There is, however, another important sense in which politics has shaped responses to the epidemic in South Africa. Gauri and Lieberman – amongst others – make a compelling set of arguments concerning the impact of racialised vectors of HIV transmission. The demographics of the epidemic in South Africa are such that HIV seroprevalence differs dramatically across race lines and between social classes. In particular, it is concentrated in the ranks of black South Africans and, initially at least, disproportionately affected the poor, unemployed and unskilled. Here, the stigmatising and 'race-based accounts of who had the disease' profoundly shaped political responses to the epidemic: first, under the white minority government (who associated the epidemic with white homosexuals and black 'terrorists') and, subsequently, under the ANC [with the prevalence of a range of conspiracy theories among the black population, and perceptions within the white population that this was a 'black' disease (Fassin and Schneider 2003; Gauri and Lieberman 2006)]. The history of colonialism and apartheid, racist population control policies and the role played by the white medical profession on South African mines, in the apartheid prisons, and the army, made South Africa ripe for the reception of conspiracy theories about the malignity of Western medicine and science (Fassin and Schneider 2003).

Consequently, 'South African political actors – high-level government leaders, church leaders, ordinary citizens – have portrayed HIV/AIDS as a problem for "them", not "us" (Gauri and Lieberman 2006).[40] This complex nexus of issues profoundly and tragically shaped the response of the government – and it seems highly likely that it has affected businesses' response too. Dickinson and Stevens, for example, argue that 'social distance between management and workers, as a result of class, race and gender, has had an important role in obscuring the view of company decision-makers as to the impact of the disease' (Dickinson and Stevens 2005). These unhappy political dynamics have severely compromised the capacity of a range of South African actors – in both the public and private sectors – to respond with the necessary speed or scale to the crisis.

Conclusion

In South Africa, the political impact of the epidemic, and what it reveals about the country's governance, has not been what one might have expected. For complex reasons, the country's democratically elected government has failed to develop an effective public sector response to the epidemic – and this has created the context within which other national actors have responded. There have been some potentially helpful responses to the epidemic from within civil society (and in particular from NGOs like the Treatment Action Campaign and dozens of smaller community-based responses) and from certain elements of the business community. Nonetheless, the failure of the South African government to develop and implement an effective HIV/AIDS programme confounds common sense expectations about the relationship between democracy, good governance and political responsiveness by the state to the epidemic.

The implications of these developments potentially reach well beyond the issue of HIV/AIDS. When seen alongside the impact of 20-odd years of neoliberal policy pressure, the epidemic may be further undermining an ideal that many still hold dear – namely that the state ought to be the primary provider of health and welfare services in society. This ideal had long been very far from the reality of the state's role in apartheid South Africa. While the ANC-led government had made important progress in providing far wider access to healthcare in the 'new' South Africa, its bungling of the HIV/AIDS response has seriously damaged both its reputation and its actual capacity to meet all of the healthcare needs of its citizenry.

Developments in South Africa also challenge minimalist conceptions of business' social responsibilities. Dickinson and Innes point out that '[a]ttempts to delimit company responsibility can be made by demarcating the respective roles of business and government – with government responsible for everything beyond the companies' gates.' They continue to note, however, that 'if HIV/AIDS is fuelled by poverty, such a division is wishful thinking' (Dickinson and Innes 2004). Business' response, however, to the socially-embedded nature of the epidemic has been, at best, partial.

Moreover, while there is no question that it is important to galvanise all possible resources to combat the epidemic, there are potentially far-reaching implications in having non-democratically elected political institutions – such as business and NGOs – delivering a significant share of those resources. There is growing evidence that the response by NGOs, whatever its implications for good governance, provides only patchy access to treatment. Similarly, while greater levels of CSR are to be welcomed, the response by the private sector is strikingly uneven and frequently rooted in self-interest. Even within those firms that offer access to ARVs for their employees, there are considerable inconsistencies in employees' actual access to those drugs and to broader medical aid insurance (Dickinson and Innes 2004). At best the latter response only addresses in a very selective manner, a tiny proportion of the workers employed in the formal sector. Moreover, as Dickinson and Innes warn:

> (w)hile nearly all large companies report having HIV/AIDS policies, many have not conducted research on what to base these policies on, programmes are often incomplete when measured against codes of good practice, there are gaps in the provision of ARV drugs to full-time employees, and there is little independent monitoring of policy implementation.
>
> (Dickinson and Innes 2004: 47)

Finally, we need also to consider very carefully what the implications are of healthcare access being provided on the basis of someone's status as a worker, rather than their status as a citizen. In the ongoing reorganisation of governance that is going on in South Africa and across the continent, universal access to healthcare is no longer secured by virtue of citizenship (and arguably never was). Even for the lucky minority who are employed in the formal sector and have the good fortune to work for an employer who has developed a comprehensive and constructive response to the epidemic, troubling questions remain: what, for example, are the implications for the right to strike, when one's employer is also the source of one's livesaving drug treatment? Similarly, what happens when a worker on an ARV course of treatment is retrenched or retires? More broadly speaking, when businesses take on some of the responsibilities for responding to the healthcare needs of their workers, does this let the state off the hook, reducing important and necessary pressure that would otherwise be directed toward fixing the state's response? There are few clear answers to these questions. In the end, there may be few acceptable substitutes for a concerted and universal state response; the dilemma for South Africans is how to proceed when their state is not ideally situated to provide such a response.

Notes

1 I would like to acknowledge the School of Public and Development Management at the University of the Witwatersrand, Johannesburg, and its director, Francis Antonie, for greatly facilitating the preliminary research for this paper. Amy Patterson provided helpful comment on an earlier draft of this chapter and a fellowship from the Comparative Program on Health and Society at the Munk Centre for International Studies at the University of Toronto subsequently provided me with crucial time and space for revisions. My thanks to them all.

2 POLICY Project *et al.*, *The Level of Effort in the National Response to HIV/AIDS: The AIDS Programme Effort Index (API) 2003 Round* (The Futures Group International, 2003 [cited September 13 2006]).

3 On the broader question of the impact of neo-liberal policies on African economies, see Thandika Mkandawire and Charles Soludo, *Our Continent, Our Future: African Perspectives on Structural Adjustment* (Asmara, Eritrea: CODESRIA, 1999) and Nicolas van de Walle, *African Economies and the Politcs of Permanent Crisis 1979–99* (Cambridge: Cambridge University Press, 2001) among many others.

4 See Global Business Coalition on HIV/AIDS, *Why Is HIV/AIDS a Business Issue?* (Global Business Coalition, [cited 16 August 2005]); available from www.businessfightsaids.org. Jonathan L Simon et al., "The Response of African Businesses to HIV/AIDS," in *HIV/AIDS in the Commonwealth 2000/01* (London: Kensington Publication, 2000).

5 There are many accounts of this. See for example Anthony Butler, "South Africa's HIV/AIDS Policy, 1994–2004: How Can It Be Explained?" *African Affairs* 104, no. 417 (2005), Didier Fassin, *When Bodies Remember: Experiences and Politics of AIDS in South Africa* (Berkeley, CA: University of California Press, 2007), and Pieter Fourie, *The Political Management of HIV and AIDS in South Africa: One Burden Too Many?* (New York: Palgrave Macmillan, 2006).

6 On this, see especially Didier Fassin and Helen Schneider, "The Politics of AIDS in Africa: Beyond the Controversies," *British Medical Journal* 326 (2003), Nicoli Nattrass, *The Moral Economy of AIDS in Southern Africa* (Cambridge: Cambridge University Press, 2004).

7 See Patrick Bond, *Elite Transition: From Apartheid to Neo-Liberalism in South Africa* (London: Pluto Press, 2000), Jonathan Michie and Vishnu Padayachee, (eds), *The Political Economy of South Africa's Transition* (London: The Dryden Press, 1997), Nicoli Nattrass, "The ANC's Economic Policy: A Critical Perspective," in *Wealth or Poverty: Critical Choices for South Africa*, (ed. Robert Schrire) (Cape Town: Oxford University Press, 1992).

8 It is one of ghastlier ironies of the new South Africa that the country's transition to democracy coincided almost entirely with the period when the incidence of transmission of HIV was accelerating most dangerously. It was also a period when business was being forced to adjust to a much more liberalised trading environment and many of the country's larger firms began to streamline and reoganise their core areas of business in order to remain competitive.

9 See http://www.sabcoha.org/who-we-are/who-we-are.html [accessed October 29, 2007] and see http://www.businessfightsaids.org [accessed January 20th, 2008].

10 Granted, it is very difficult to distinguish between job-shedding as a result of the epidemic, and job-shedding that is simply part of the restructuring of labour: capital ratios by business in the neo-liberal era.

11 D Dickinson and M Stevens, "Understanding the Response of Large South African Companies to HIV/AIDS," *Journal of Social Aspects of HIV/AIDS* 2, no. 2 (2005): 288. Firms are, of course, obliged to apply the existing legal framework in how they treat their employees. For example, they are not allowed to discriminate on the basis of HIV status. Firms are also encouraged to adopt the best practice laid out in NEDLAC, *Code of Good Practice on Key Aspects of HIV/AIDS and Employment* (National Economic Development Labour Council, 2000 [cited 30 November 2007]); available from http://www.nedlac.org.za/top.asp?inc=docs/agreements/code_aids.html. However the law does not directly require any systematic or proactive programme for the workplace. David Dickinson and Duncan Innes, "Fronts or Front-Lines? HIV/AIDS and Big Business in South Africa," *Transformation* 55 (2004): 31.

12 This also assumes that firms have relatively accurate information about what that impact is likely to be. Larger firms will obviously be at an advantage here because of their in-house research capacity. Personal correspondence with Amy Patterson.

13 See Thomas W Dunfee, "Do Firms with Unique Competencies for Rescuing Victims of Human Catastrophes Have Special Obligations? Corporate Responsibility and the AIDS Catastrophe in Sub-Saharan Africa," *Business Ethics Quarterly* 16, no. 2 (2006), Martha L Salomon, "AIDS Is Risky Business: Examining the Effect of the AIDS Crisis on Publicly Traded Companies in South Africa and the Implications for Both South African and U.S. Investors," *Vanderbilt Journal of Transnational Law* 37 (2004).

14 Pressure groups here might include trade unions, activist consumer groups and certain churches. (The reaction by churches has been almost as variegated and diverse as the response of the broader population more generally.)

15 For a discussion of path dependency analyses, see for example James Mahoney, "Path Dependence in Historical Sociology," *Theory and Society* 29, no. 4 (2000), Paul Pierson, "Increasing Returns, Path Dependency and the Study of Politics," *American Political Science Review* 94, no. 2 (2002).

16 These findings are based on fieldwork undertaken in South African and Uganda respectively in the summer of 2006. In each instance I interviewed 20–30 people in both business and government circles about the macro-economic impact of the epidemic and the consequences of this for their own strategic thinking and planning.

17 See discussion of SABCOHA survey in Dickinson and Innes, 'Fronts or Front-Lines? HIV/AIDS and Big Business in South Africa'

18 See Bureau for Economic Research, 'The Macroeconomic Impact of HIV/AIDS Under Alternative Intervention Scenarios (with Specific Reference to ART) on the South African Economy' (Stellenbosch, South Africa: Bureau for Economic Research, University of Stellenbosch, 2006).

19 By contrast, when I was in Uganda for my pilot study, this task had barely begun: The Ugandan AIDS Commission had just commissioned precisely such a study and a team was in the preliminary stages of setting this up but no projections were as yet available. Little research – or direction – is coming from Ugandan business associations either. When I visited the Private Sector Foundation, I met with several of their senior staff. When I asked what the impact of the epidemic was on their members, they responded that they could not say precisely and added that 'it would be a good idea if somebody did a study of that.' As a result, decision makers in firms must instead plan and make judgments based on anecdotal evidence and their own social and firm-level experiences.

20 They have funded a good deal of research. See for example Kristina Quattek, "The Economic Impact of AIDS in South Africa: A Dark Cloud on the Horizon," in

Konrad Adenauer Stiftung Occasional Papers (Johannesburg, South Africa: ING Barings, 2000).

21 See for example Unattributed, "Live the Future: HIV and AIDS Scenarios for South Africa: 2005–25," (Belville, South Africa: Metropolitan, 2005), and Alan Whiteside and Clem Sunter, *AIDS: The Challenge for South Africa* (Johannesburg, South Africa: Human and Rosseau, 2000).

22 As with the prognosis for the continent more broadly, so too in South Africa do economists differ wildly in their projections of the impact of the epidemic on the broader economy. For a lucid overview of the various models, see Nattrass, *The Moral Economy of AIDS in Southern Africa*.

23 South Africa's epidemic, like others on the sub-continent, has afflicted high numbers of women. There is some debate about why this is but most agree that women are not only physiologically more susceptible to the virus than men, but gendered socio-economic inequalities, including lower levels of income, formal employment and education and in some cases difficulties in negotiating the terms of sexual relationships probably also contribute to their vulnerability. Anne V Akeroyd, "Coercion, Constraints and 'Cultural Entrapments': A Further Look at Gendered and Occupational Factors Pertinent to the Transmission of HIV in Africa," in *HIV and AIDS in Africa: Beyond Epidemiology*, ed. Ezekiel Kalipeni *et al.* (Oxford: Blackwell Publishing, 2004).

24 Most of those sick and dying are unskilled; or at least this was true for a long time. There is growing evidence of prevalence in white collar workers, including in the public sector, within the ranks of nurses, policeofficers, and teachers. N Nattrass, "AIDS, Growth and Distribution in South Africa," in *Centre for Social Science Research Working Paper No. 7* (Cape Town, South Africa: University of Cape Town, 2002).

25 It bears remarking that the analysis may also be fundamentally misconceived. For a start, this view ignores the complex interdependencies between the formal and informal economies, not to mention considering that, in the medium-to long-term, the social and political toll of the disease is unlikely to leave the broader economy unscathed. See the arguments in Channing Arndt and Jeffrey D. Lewis, "The HIV/AIDS Pandemic in South Africa: Sectoral Impacts and Unemployment," *Journal of International Development* 13 (2001) and Richard Devey, Caroline Skinner and Imraan Valodia, "Second Best? Trends and Linkages in the Informal Economy in South Africa," *DPRU Working Paper* no. 06/102 (February 2006).

26 By contrast in Uganda, the epidemic reaches much more evenly into the society; thus significant numbers of both skilled and unskilled workers – at the very heart of the economy – have been affected.

27 H Bhorat and Johan Hodge, "Decomposing Shifts in Labour Demand in South Africa," *South African Journal of Economics* 67, no. 3 (1999), pp. 155–68. There is some contention over the reasons for this shift. Bhorat and Hodge consider changes in methods of production that contributed: unionisation, they argue, and subsequent increases in the wages of unskilled labour after the mid 1970s shifted relative prices in favour of capital. However, they conclude that the key factor shaping the changing labour demand patterns in South Africa has been the adoption of new technology (especially microelectronics) as services has grown to become one of the key sectors in the economy. This has further heightened the demand for skilled workers and decreased the demand for the unskilled.

28 While previous epidemics may have boosted the power of labour, it must be remembered that South Africa currently suffers from a significant *oversupply* of unskilled labour. If the epidemic does indeed make the use of labour more expensive (or even just more troublesome in the minds of employers), it may exacerbate the already existing tendency of employers to substitute capital for labour, thus eradicating more jobs. These dynamics can inspire grisly calculations. In the end of

course, should very large numbers of workers die, this will ultimately shift the value of labour, but at the moment, it seems that the oversupply of unskilled labour still outweighs the impact of AIDS deaths.

29 See for example World Economic Forum, "Anglogold," in *Gobal Health Initiative: Private Sector Intervention Case Example* (Geneva, Switzerland: World Economic Forum, Undated), World Economic Forum, "Gold Fields Limited," in *Global Health Initiative: Private Sector Intervention Case Example* (Geneva, Switzerland: World Economic Forum, Undated).

30 Ahwireng-Obeng at al argue that construction has been affected principally via "increases in costs related to training and recruiting, replacement employees and funeral costs." Cited in Meintjes, Bowen, and Root, "HIV/AIDS in the South African Construction Industry: Understanding the HIV/AIDS Discourse for a Sector-Specific Response," 259. See also "The impact of HIV/AIDS on selected business sectors in South Africa 2005", SABCOHA and Bureau for Economic Research, 2005.

31 Personal communication with Stephen Lehrer.
Indications are moreover that the mining industry calculated that the costs imposed on them by the epidemic would be substantial, adding as much as $10 to the price of an ounce of gold. Michael Dynes, "GoldFields' Estimate of AIDS Costs Highlights Economic Costs of Epidemic," *The Star,* 9 April 2002.

32 Fourie describes how NUM "focused on the deleterious effect that the migrant labour system was having in spreading the epidemic. Rather than repatriation [of miners to their villages], the NUM called for a human rights approach, insisting that counselling and adequate health facilities, as well as follow-up facilities, be provided for HIV-positive workers. Furthermore, the NUM called for compensation for workers whose working lives had been cut short by the disease." Fourie, *The Political Management of HIV and AIDS in South Africa: One Burden Too Many?* 82. The unions approach was not always this constructive. In the early days of the epidemic, key union officials did not want to address the issue for fear it would play into racist stereotypes about black sexual promiscuity.

33 A historical precedent in this regard was set by the leadership provided by the same few large mining companies in shaping the overall sub-sector's responses to its broader political context, for example the industry's relationship with the apartheid government and, following the legalisation of trade unions, the evolving relationship with labour. A number of authors highlight the role of "peer pressure" from other firms in their study. Cf. Dickinson and Stevens, "Understanding the Response of Large South African Companies to HIV/AIDS", Dickinson and Innes, "Fronts or Front-Lines? HIV/AIDS and Big Business in South Africa."

34 In a survey of South Africa's 50 largest firms, the top two reasons cited for motivating the company's response to HIV/AIDS were, first, the need "to act as a responsible corporate citizen," and, second, concern about the economic impact of the epidemic on the firm. Dickinson and Innes, "Fronts or Front-Lines? HIV/AIDS and Big Business in South Africa," 39.

35 The same trend has been evident in the South African garment manufacturing industry; these companies too (like construction) have been strikingly unresponsive in their responses to the AIDS epidemic.

36 For more on the important role of pan-business organisation, and how this shapes business-government relations, see Antoinette Handley, *Business and the State in Africa: Economic Policymaking in the Neo-Liberal Era* (London: Cambridge University Press, Forthcoming), Ben Ross Schneider, "Why Is Mexican Business So Organized?" *Latin American Research Review* 37, no. 1 (2002).

37 It is less clear why the mining industry has not challenged the government more forthrightly, given the significant costs that the epidemic poses for mining and this sector's relative independence from government. One can only speculate it was

somehow less palatable for the mining industry to confront Mbeki's government on this issue than to simply deal with the matter internally.

38 Stephen Clarkson has suggested that this difference may have to do with customer base. Commercial banks have branches in even the smallest communities and many of their customers are individual South Africans. They are therefore reminded on a daily basis of the impact of epidemic on the broader population, and on their customers. IT firms, by contrast, tend to mostly serve other companies. Their daily contact with their customers will also tend to be with highly skilled and educated people – where prevalence levels are lower. Personal communication with Stephen Clarkson.

39 It is striking that Chamber of Mines, by contrast, was relatively assertive in challenging the white minority government in 1989 for "not taking the threat posed by AIDS seriously enough." Fourie, *The Political Management of HIV and AIDS in South Africa: One Burden Too Many?* 82.

40 Friedman and Mottiar describe how in the 1980s, the union active in the mining sector resisted early calls to address the issue for fear that this would feed into racist stereotypes about black sexuality. Steven Friedman and Shauna Mottiar, "A Rewarding Engagement? The Treatment Action Campaign and the Politics of HIV/AIDS," *Politics and Society* 33, no. 4 (2005).

Bibliography

Akeroyd, A.V. (2004). 'Coercion, Constraints and "Cultural Entrapments": A Further Look at Gendered and Occupational Factors Pertinent to the Transmission of HIV in Africa' in *HIV and AIDS in Africa: Beyond Epidemiology*, edited by Ezekiel Kalipeni, Susan Craddock, Joseph R Oppong and Jayati Ghosh, 89–103. Oxford: Blackwell Publishing.

Allen, T. and S. Heald. (2004). 'HIV/AIDS Policy in Africa: What Has Worked in Uganda and What Has Failed in Botswana?' *Journal of International Development* 16: 1141–54.

Arndt, C. and Lewis, J.D. (2001). 'The HIV/AIDS Pandemic in South Africa: Sectoral Impacts and Unemployment' *Journal of International Development* 13: 427–49.

Barnett, T. and Whiteside, A. (2002). *AIDS in the Twenty-First Century: Disease and Globalization*. Pietermaritzburg, South Africa: Palgrave Macmillan.

Bendell, J. (2003). 'Waking up to Risk: Corporate Responses to HIV/AIDS in the Workplace' edited by UNRISD Programme on Technology, Business and Society and Joint UN Programme on HIV/AIDS: United Nations Research Institute for Social Development.

Bhorat, H. and Hodge, J. (1999). 'Decomposing Shifts in Labour Demand in South Africa' *South African Journal of Economics* 67(3): 155–68.

Bond, P. (2000). *Elite Transition: From Apartheid to Neo-Liberalism in South Africa*. London: Pluto Press.

Bor, J. (2007). 'The Political Economy of AIDS Leadership in Developing Countries: An Exploratory Analysis' *Social Science and Medicine* 64(8): 1585–99.

Bureau for Economic Research. (2006). 'The Macroeconomic Impact of HIV/AIDS under Alternative Intervention Scenarios (with Specific Reference to ART) on the South African Economy' 139. Stellenbosch, South Africa: Bureau for Economic Research, University of Stellenbosch.

Butler, A. (2005). 'South Africa's HIV/AIDS Policy, 1994–2004: How Can It Be Explained?' *African Affairs* 104(417): 591–614.

Devey, R, Skinner, R. and Valodia, I. (2006). 'Second Best? Trends and Linkages in the Informal Economy in South Africa' *DPRU Working Paper* no. 06/102

De Waal, A. (2006). *AIDS and Power: Why There Is No Political Crisis – Yet.* London: Zed Books.

Dickinson, D, and Stevens, M. (2005). 'Understanding the Response of Large South African Companies to HIV/AIDS' *Journal of Social Aspects of HIV/AIDS* 2(2): 286–95.

Dickinson, D. and Innes, D. (2004). 'Fronts or Front-Lines? HIV/AIDS and Big Business in South Africa' *Transformation* 55: 28–54.

Dixon, S., McDonald, S. and Roberts, J. (2001). 'AIDS and Economic Growth in Africa: A Panel Data Analysis' *Journal of International Development* 13: 411–26.

Drummond, D. and Kelly, R. (2006). 'The Economic Cost of AIDS: A Clear Case for Action' 14: TD Economics

Dunfee, R.W. (2006). 'Do Firms with Unique Competencies for Rescuing Victims of Human Catastrophes Have Special Obligations? Corporate Responsibility and the AIDS Catastrophe in Sub-Saharan Africa.' *Business Ethics Quarterly* 16(2): 185–210.

Dynes, M. (2002). 'GoldFields' Estimate of AIDS Costs Highlights Economic Costs of Epidemic' *The Star*, 9 April.

Epstein, H. (2007). *The Invisible Cure: Africa, the West and the Fight against AIDS* New York: Farrar, Straus and Giroux.

Evans, P.B. (1995). *Embedded Autonomy: States and Industrial Transformation.* Princeton, NJ: Princeton University Press.

Fassin, D. (2007). *When Bodies Remember: Experiences and Politics of AIDS in South Africa.* Berkeley, CA: University of California Press.

Fassin, D. and Schneider, H. (2003). 'The Politics of AIDS in Africa: Beyond the Controversies' *British Medical Journal* 326: 495–97.

Fourie, P. (2006). *The Political Management of HIV and AIDS in South Africa: One Burden Too Many?* New York: Palgrave Macmillan

Friedman, M. (1970). 'A Friedman Doctrine – the Social Responsibility of Business Is to Increase Its Profits' *The New York Times Magazine*, September 13, 122–26.

Friedman, S. and Mottiar, S. (2005). 'A Rewarding Engagement? The Treatment Action Campaign and the Politics of HIV/AIDS' *Politics and Society* 33(4): 511–65.

Gauri, V. and Lieberman, E.S. (2006). 'Boundary Institutions and HIV/AIDS Policy in Brazil and South Africa.' *Studies in Comparative International Development* 41 (3): 47–73.

Global Business Coalition on HIV/AIDS. (2005). 'Why Is HIV/AIDS a Business Issue?' in, Global Business Coalition, www.businessfightsaids.org. (accessed 16 August, 2005).

Granovetter, M. (1985). 'Economic Action and Social Structure: The Problem of Embeddedness' *American Journal of Sociology* 91(3)

Handley, A. (forthcoming). *Business and the State in Africa: Economic Policymaking in the Neo-Liberal Era.* London: Cambridge University Press,

—— (2005). 'Business, Government and Economic Policymaking in the New South Africa, 1990–2000' *Journal of Modern African Studies* 43(2): 211–39.

—— (2004). 'The New South Africa, a Decade Later' *Current History* 103(673): 195–201.

Mahoney, J. (2000). 'Path Dependence in Historical Sociology' *Theory and Society* 29 (4): 507–48.

Maxfield, S., and Schneider, B.R. (1997). *Business and the State in Developing Countries.* Ithaca, NY: Cornell University Press.

McGregor, B.F.A (2004). *McGregor's Who Owns Whom in South Africa*, 24th edn Florida Hills, South Africa: Carla Soares.

Meintjes, I., Bowen, P. and Root, D. (2007). 'HIV/AIDS in the South African Construction Industry: Understanding the HIV/AIDS Discourse for a Sector-Specific Response' *Construction Management and Economics* 25(3): 255–66.

Michie, J. and Padayachee, R. (eds) (1997). *The Political Economy of South Africa's Transition*. London: The Dryden Press.

Mkandawire, T. and Soludo, C. (1999). *Our Continent, Our Future: African Perspectives on Structural Adjustment*. Asmara, Eritrea: CODESRIA.

Nabila, J.S., Antwi, P., Yeboah, K. and Kwankye, S. (2001). 'A Study of the Economic Impact of HIV/AIDS on Selected Business Organizations in Ghana' 37. Accra, Ghana: POLICY Project, 2001.

Nattrass, N. (2004). *The Moral Economy of AIDS in Southern Africa*: Cambridge University Press.

—— (2002). 'AIDS, Growth and Distribution in South Africa' In *Centre for Social Science Research Working Paper No. 7*. Cape Town, South Africa: University of Cape Town.

—— (1992). 'The ANC's Economic Policy: A Critical Perspective' in *Wealth or Poverty: Critical Choices for South Africa*, edited by Robert Schrire. Cape Town: Oxford University Press.

Nattrass, N., Neilson, T. Bery, P., Mistry, N. and Sievers, S.E. (2005). 'Opportunities for Business in the Fight against HIV/AIDS' Global Business Coalition on HIV/AIDS.

NEDLAC. (2000). 'Code of Good Practice on Key Aspects of HIV/AIDS and Employment' in National Economic Development Labour Council, http://www.nedlac.org.za/top.asp?inc=docs/agreements/code_aids.html. (accessed 30 November, 2007).

Patterson, A.S. (ed.) (2005). *The African State and the AIDS Crisis.* Aldershot, Hants UK: Ashgate

Pierson, P. (2002). 'Increasing Returns, Path Dependency and the Study of Politics' *American Political Science Review* 94(2): 251–67.

Poku, N.K, and Whiteside, A. (eds) (2004). *The Political Economy of AIDS in Africa.* Aldershot, Hants UK: Ashgate.

Policy Coordination and Advisory Services; The Presidency. (2004). 'Towards a Ten Year Review: Synthesis Report on Implementation of Government Programmes' Pretoria, South Africa: Government Communications.

POLICY Project, USAID, UNAIDS, and WHO. (2003). The Level of Effort in the National Response to HIV/AIDS: The AIDS Programme Effort Index (API) 2003 Round. In, The Futures Group International (Accessed September 13, 2006).

Putzel, J. (2004). 'The Politics of Action on AIDS: A Case Study of Uganda' *Public Administration and Development* 24(1): 19–30.

Quattek, K. (2000). 'The Economic Impact of AIDS in South Africa: A Dark Cloud on the Horizon' in *Konrad Adenauer Stiftung Occasional Papers.* Johannesburg, South Africa: ING Barings

Rhodes, R.A.W. (1996). 'The New Governance: Governing without Government' *Political Studies* XLIV: 652–67.

Rosen, S. and Simon, J.L. (2003). 'Shifting the Burden: The Private Sector's Response to the Aids Epidemic in Africa' *Bulletin of the World Health Organization* 81(2): 131–37.

Salomon, M.L. (2004). 'AIDS Is Risky Business: Examining the Effect of the AIDS Crisis on Publicly Traded Companies in South Africa and the Implications for Both South African and U.S. Investors' *Vanderbilt Journal of Transnational Law* 37: 1473–1509.

Schneider, B.R. (2004). *Business Politics and the State in Twentieth-Century Latin America*. Cambridge: Cambridge University Press.

—— (2002). 'Why Is Mexican Business So Organized?' *Latin American Research Review* 37(1): 77–118.

Simon, J.L, Rosen, S., Whiteside, A., Vincent, J.R., and Thea, D.M. (2000). 'The Response of African Businesses to HIV/AIDS' in *HIV/AIDS in the Commonwealth 2000/01*. London: Kensington Publication.

UNAIDS. (2006). 'Report on the Global AIDS Epidemic.'

Unattributed. (2005). "Live the Future: HIV and AIDS Scenarios for South Africa: 2005–25." 25. Belville, South Africa: Metropolitan.

van de Walle, N.(2001). *African Economies and the Politcs of Permanent Crisis 1979–99*. Cambridge: Cambridge University Press.

Vogel, D. (2005). *The Market for Virtue: The Potential and Limits of Corporate Social Responsibility*. Washington D.C.: Brookings Institution Press.

Whiteside, A. and Sunter, C. (2000). *AIDS: The Challenge for South Africa*. Johannesburg, South Africa: Human and Rosseau.

World Economic Forum. (2002) 'Anglogold' in *Global Health Initiative: Private Sector Intervention Case Example*, 8. Geneva, Switzerland: World Economic Forum, Undated.

——. 'Gold Fields Limited' In *Global Health Initiative: Private Sector Intervention Case Example*, 7. Geneva, Switzerland: World Economic Forum, Undated.

Youde, J. (2007). *AIDS, South Africa, and the Politics of Knowledge*. Aldershot: Ashgate

6 The private sector and governance of the HIV/AIDS response

Franklyn Lisk

HIV/AIDS is a global epidemic that is crippling economies and markets around the world, particularly in Sub-Saharan Africa, which is the hardest hit region. According to UNAIDS, an estimated 33 million people worldwide were living with HIV in 2007, and the epidemic has already claimed the lives of over 25 million people (UNAIDS and WHO 2007; UNAIDS 2008). In many developing countries, HIV infection is concentrated in the working-age population and those in the prime of their productive lives (15–49 years). The International Labour Organisation (ILO) estimates that over three-quarters of those living with HIV are persons of working age, which implies that most of those who have died from AIDS-related illnesses came from the workforce, whether employed or unemployed (ILO/AIDS 2004 and ILO/AIDS 2006). The impact of AIDS on the workforce results in losses both in the quantity and quality of labour and, consequently, declining productivity and increasing costs in production. HIV/AIDS is recognised by the ILO and its tripartite constituents[1] in the organisation's code of practice for dealing with the epidemic in the workplace as a 'workplace issue' (ILO 2001), on account of its effect on the workforce and the potentially devastating impact of the epidemic on enterprises.

Losses in labour supply and productivity pose an exceptional challenge for the private sector, where the survival of a business depends crucially on its workforce as its most important asset. In addition to the direct costs of AIDS-related morbidity and mortality to enterprise, there are indirect costs that are linked to productivity losses and higher than normal output costs which impact negatively on enterprise performance. AIDS-related absenteeism – due to illness of workers, time taken off work to care for sick family members and to attend funerals – could reduce profits and investments, and contribute to loss of competitiveness in domestic and international markets. By the start of the new millennium, there was sufficient evidence that HIV/AIDS was adversely affecting productivity and the output and delivery of goods and services in manufacturing and agricultural enterprises in highly-affected countries in southern and eastern Africa (Greener 1997; McPherson *et al.* 2000; Hacker 2001; Rosen *et al.* 2003). Some employers in South Africa, Botswana, Swaziland, Uganda and Kenya had already realised the threat of

HIV/AIDS to business and, accordingly, introduced specific measures to address this threat to their companies (Cohen 1998; Bonnel 2000, 2001; UNAIDS 2005).

This chapter is about the response of the private sector to the HIV/AIDS epidemic and governance. Based on a growing body of evidence from national experiences that effective governance is essential for an effective response to the epidemic (Roderick 2004; Lisk 2006c; UNDP 2007), it focuses on the types of interventions adopted by firms and business organisations to deal with the impact of HIV/AIDS on the private sector, and how these interventions contribute to improved governance. The chapter begins with an overview of the impact of HIV/AIDS on the private sector, highlighting how the epidemic affects the interests of the private sector, both business and labour alike. It then presents and analyses the response of the private sector: explaining how and why firms decide to provide HIV/AIDS services to their employees and the local community, including an analysis of the costs to business and the benefits that can be derived from such interventions; and identifying the governance implications of the workplace strategies, policies and programmes adopted, the private sector to respond to the epidemic. The case studies selected have chosen to illustrate how firms have been able to apply the principles promoted in the ILO Code of Practice on HIV/AIDS and the World of Work (ILO 2001)

Impact of HIV/AIDS on the private sector

The impact of the HIV/AIDS epidemic on the private sector will depend on a number of factors, such as the HIV prevalence rate in a country, the capital: labour ratio in production and the extent to which the government is committed and actually takes action against the spread of HIV in the country. It has been noted that the cost of HIV/AIDS to an enterprise could be as high as 10–20 per cent of annual labour cost in a private sector business (UNDP/Government of Malawi 2002; Vass 2005; Whiteside 2008). This massive increase in production costs in key sectors, and the effects on profits and corporate tax revenues, combine to undermine economic growth and progress towards long-term sustainable development. Such is the concern of the United Nations (UN) and the international community about this wider development impact of the global HIV/AIDS epidemic, that control of the spread of the HIV was declared one of the eight Millennium Development Goals (MDGs)[2], which were established in the Declaration adopted by the UN Millennium Summit in September 2000 (UN 2000).

The private sector, including subsistence agriculture and the urban informal economy, is the main provider of employment opportunities in many developing countries, including those most affected by HIV/AIDS. Labour losses in the private sector due to HIV/AIDS include skilled workers and a range of capacities that may be undervalued by conventional classification. Tasks that can be classified as 'organisational' – e.g. those undertaken by supervisory workers and management staff, who often play key roles in production and whose skills derive from years of experience – are particularly relevant. The probability is that losses of key personnel with job-specific skills and organisational experience will disrupt production and diminish product/service quality. As already noted, firms are affected not only through the direct effects of absenteeism/sickness and related disruption of production on costs, which limit the ability of employers to retain a stable workforce; they also have to incur additional indirect costs to support viable health insurance and pension schemes for the benefit of workers who fall ill and retire prematurely, and to recruit and train new staff. Profits of firms could shrink as a result of the direct and indirect costs of HIV/AIDS production and the loss of markets due to widespread AIDS-related deaths among the general population.

Such had been the impact of AIDS on firms in the private sector that by the mid-1990s, larger firms in some of the worst hit countries were no longer seeking to justify their involvement by asking, 'Why should we respond?', but instead wanted answers to questions such as 'How should we respond?', 'What should we do?' and, 'Who can we work with?' Compelling evidence of the direct and indirect costs of HIV/AIDS to business emerged from a number of empirical studies on the impact of the epidemic on labour productivity and costs (Rosen, *et al* 2003; Natrass, *et al.* 2005) helped to convince the private sector employers that on balance there is a good business case for providing comprehensive HIV/AIDS services to their employees. The determinants of decisions by enterprises to provide HIV/AIDS services are influenced largely by an assessment of the impact of HIV/AIDS on the firm's productivity and production costs in relation to the costs to the firm of providing such services, sickness benefits and recruitment/training of new workers. Because of the costs involved in providing HIV/AIDS services, workplace programmes have been dominated by transnational corporations and larger enterprises whose resource base and institutional capacity enable them to undertake comprehensive action against the epidemic. A study by the Washington think-tank, Center for Global Development (CDG), which analysed data from 860 firms and 4,955 workers in Kenya,Tanzania and Uganda, found that larger firms and those with more highly skilled workers invested more in HIV/AIDS prevention and treatment (Ramachandran *et al.* 2006).

Costs and benefits of HIV/AIDS interventions in the private sector

Calculating the costs of the HIV/AIDS epidemic to business has not been easy or straightforward, because of lack of data, the array of different factors to be measured and the many assumptions about what and how to measure. There are direct and indirect costs and costs that are specific to an individual firm or industry, etc. Some of the more severe costs of HIV/AIDS cannot be measured by quantifiable measurement techniques. The complexity of calculating the costs of HIV/AIDS affects the determination of what can be incorporated in a cost–benefit analysis. For the sake of simplicity, we can assume that companies incur costs and expect to derive benefits when they invest in the provision of HIV/AIDS prevention, treatment and care in the workplace. This implies that the aim of preventative action in the workplace is to reduce the number of employees who will get infected, while treatment programmes are designed to extend the working life of employees already infected.

In the absence of treatment and care, workers who are HIV-positive are likely to fall ill and be absent from work more frequently than usual. The chances are that in highly affected countries anywhere from 20 to 60 per cent of a company's workforce may be infected with and/or affected by HIV/AIDS. Without treatment, almost all of the infected workers will die sooner or later – and well before they reach retirement age. Furthermore, as noted, employers may have to pay out death-related benefits to surviving dependents and/or contribute to funeral expenses. On top of these, employers may also have to incur additional costs in relation to recruitment and training of replacement workers, which can be quite high in a labour market that is already constrained by shortages of skilled workers. Disruptions to production due to absenteeism, and pressure on the remaining workers to maintain production, could undermine morale as well as contribute to deterioration in labour relations within a firm. Supervisors and management could spend their time dealing with AIDS-related workplace problems, including arranging funerals and addressing discrimination and stigma, rather than their normal duties, resulting in a decline in production and efficiency.

The integration of HIV/AIDS services into established occupational health and safety programmes makes good business sense, as it can reduce the cost of interventions as well as help to address problems of stigma and discrimination in the workplace. The private sector gains from corporate involvement and investment in prevention and treatment, in the sense that work is maintained and the enterprise retains access to skills. This means that firms will face lower costs, resulting from less absenteeism and disruption of work, lower retraining costs, and higher productivity across the enterprise; skills and experience specific to the firm will also remain useful for longer. A good employer will understand this, and will ensure that personnel policy and other support services are in place to keep HIV-positive and other affected employees productive for as long as possible.

Effective response to HIV/AIDS by the private sector can generate benefits elsewhere in the economy. HIV-positive workers who receive treatment could continue to work and earn an income to support themselves and their dependents, and generate potential tax revenues on incomes and expenditures for government. In the absence of treatment, they become a burden or additional cost to the state and their families. But a comprehensive approach to the HIV/AIDS response in the workplace could be costly; even with the substantial reduction in the costs of antiretroviral (ARV) drugs, they could still be beyond the resource capabilities of many companies in developing countries (UNAIDS 2005).

Private sector response to HIV/AIDS and governance

Before the HIV/AIDS epidemic, the involvement of the private sector in promoting the workplace as a provider of healthcare had been mainly through the application of Occupational Safety and Health (OSH) standards of the ILO, which are designed to provide a safe and healthy working environment (ILO 2003). HIV/AIDS has substantially increased the amount of resources and multiplicity of skills that the private sector requires to deal with occupational health problems. The increasing involvement of the private sector in responding to the impact of HIV/AIDS in the workplace and beyond has been influenced by the exceptionality of HIV/AIDS, which makes the epidemic a wider development challenge, and by the inability of governments in some of the most affected countries to take on a larger share of the burden of HIV/AIDS on the country. The motivation for the private sector to intervene to address HIV/AIDS, and the modality of their interventions, give rise to the need to balance business interests with broader social and economic development objectives, and thus have implications for governance.

First, we need to look at the role and efficacy of private sector in promoting governance, because governance matters for effective HIV/AIDS response. Some of the interventions by the private sector, as we shall argue, are positively associated with governance, insofar as they involve measures and outcomes which: (i) facilitate local-level participation in the process and benefits of development through the expansion of HIV/AIDS services in the community; (ii) promote human rights and enhance human security through addressing stigma and discrimination, including gender biases in HIV/AIDS workplace policies and programmes; (iii) ensure efficient allocation and use of funds; (iv) encourage accountability and transparency in the HIV/AIDS response by making use of public–private partnerships and engaging civil society, particularly youth and women's organisations; and (v) strengthen cooperation with global institutions for mobilising resources and improving coordination with donors to support the HIV/AIDS efforts in developing countries.

The response of the private sector to HIV/AIDS was given a big boost worldwide with the establishment of the Global Business Council on HIV/AIDS (GBC) in 1997 (the name was later changed to the Global Business Coalition). The GBC was set up as a global umbrella organisation of businesses specifically to mobilize and channel support to the private sector response to HIV/AIDS. From the outset, the GBC emphasised the need for firms and enterprises to join forces through regional and national organisations of businesses to ward off the threat posed by HIV/AIDS to the private sector. Before the establishment of the GBC, those firms that took action against the epidemic were often working in isolation; others, even though aware of the threat of HIV/AIDS, simply did not know how to proceed. The business coalition model was developed to provide the private sector with the tools and support necessary to develop a comprehensive response to the epidemic.

The GBC has been instrumental in promoting the business coalition model among businesses worldwide, with important governance implications. GBC affiliates at regional, national and sectoral levels now include professional bodies, chambers of commerce, employer federations and even labour unions, in addition to businesses (GBC 2001; GHI/WEF 2008). Soon after it was established, the GBC launched a global campaign, which called on businesses to allocate funds for HIV/AIDS prevention, treatment and care programmes and to take action to eliminate HIV-related discrimination in the workplace. The GBC also encouraged its affiliates and their membership to work with other stakeholders, including government and civil society organisations, and to extend their HIV/AIDS services beyond the workplace and into the local community (GBC 2001; GBC 2003; WEF 2004). It warned that companies that do not address the effects of the epidemic on their business would find it hard to compete in both the domestic and global markets, and drew the attention of the private sector to the positive benefits and avoidance of costs to be derived from effective HIV/AIDS policy and programme responses (GBC 2001). At the international level, GBC has collaborated with UN agencies and other global institutions to establish international guidelines and to mobilize resources for the global HIV/AIDS response, including involvement in global and regional initiatives for substantial reductions in the price of ARV drugs.

Initially, efforts by the private sector to address HIV/AIDS were limited to the provision of services to their own employees and other measures within the workplace. For reasons linked to both business motive and corporate social responsibility (CSR), the private sector in many of the highly affected countries soon realised that it was in their interest to extend workplace HIV/AIDS services to the families of their employees and even to the local communities from which they recruited workers. However, the involvement of the private sector in extending HIV/AIDS services beyond the workplace has raised the question of how far it can go in providing healthcare for all, which is after all the responsibility of the government. The private sector's involvement in extending HIV/AIDS services to the community is a CSR issue, but one that should be viewed in the light of its core imperative of running businesses.

When the private sector invests in healthcare infrastructure and services, it is first and foremost for the benefit of their own employees. However, where there are deficits in the public provision of healthcare, the provision of services by employers in the workplace could result in the creation of 'islands of excellence' in the midst of run-down or under-resourced public sector healthcare facilities in the community. Workplace programmes offered in communities with particularly poor health infrastructure must also deal with the difficult issue that their efforts may be creating disparities in care and treatment within those communities. Essentially, employees who benefit from access to workplace-based healthcare services are better off than others in the community, which raises an equity and governance issue and underlines the need for improved access to health as a basic need and a right for all. There are reports that some workers who are benefitting from HIV/AIDS care and treatment services in the workplace have expressed concerns about the 'unfairness' of not making such services available to their wives and partners, and other members of their extended family (Lisk 2006a; Beckmann *et al.* 2005). In societies that define a family more broadly, community outreach efforts could resolve concerns that family members are excluded from accessing treatment, care and support. The ILO Code of Practice recommends that all necessary steps should be taken to ensure that workers and their families receive coverage from HIV/AIDS services. Ideally, employers' decisions to provide HIV/AIDS services to the local community need to be supported by national policies and programmes in order to secure an equitable level of healthcare in societies. Failure to link workplace community outreach HIV/AIDS programmes with government efforts may lead to increasing disparities and even social tensions.

An increasing number of transnational and larger enterprises consider it good corporate judgment to extend workplace HIV/AIDS and other health services to local communities. They have come to realise that ignoring the healthcare deprivation and poverty in the communities around them is not only bad for their corporate image, but also not good for business. The effectiveness of the HIV/AIDS response in the workplace could be diluted if interventions were not sustained between the workplace and the home and extended into the community. For example, prevention programmes in the workplace could be of little use if they were not extended to the local community in which workers live and from which they are recruited. Several HIV/AIDS workplace programmes in Africa, such as those operated by Anglo American, BHP Billiton, BMW of South Africa, Daimler-Chrysler South Africa, Eskom and Heineken International, have extended service availability to the wives and partners of their workers, which contributes towards reducing existing gender inequalities in terms of access to HIV/AIDS services (UNAIDS 2005; GBC 2003).

Public–private partnerships

Because of the high cost of providing comprehensive HIV/AIDS services, public–private partnerships (PPPs) are being used increasingly to scale up and expand prevention, treatment and care programmes. PPP is regarded as a practical arrangement for responding to demands on the private sector to extend HIV/AIDS services beyond the workplace to the local community, as well as for addressing the inability of government to provide adequate healthcare facilities and services for all. Business alone cannot absorb all the costs of providing HIV/AIDS services in the community, nor can business address HIV/AIDS as a cost issue. For this reason, Heineken International in Africa has relied on partnerships between itself and governments, NGOs, universities, UN agencies, the GBC and pharmaceutical groups, to develop its care and treatment programme. Government, the authority responsible for putting in place the regulatory and policy framework for private sector participation in the economy, is well placed to work in partnership with the private sector in AIDS response. For example, government can provide administrative, legislative and fiscal incentives to facilitate a strong private sector response to the epidemic. Private sector businesses in turn can work with government to address and share the social and health costs of HIV/AIDS, through community outreach programmes.

Partnership between the public and private sectors in HIV/AIDS response was recognised and endorsed at the June 2001 United Nations General Assembly Special Session on HIV/AIDS (UNGASS), when international business leaders joined world leaders at the UN to map out strategies and policies for an effective response to the global HIV/AIDS crisis (UN 2001). The UNGASS conclusions recognised that PPP could enhance the capacity of both business and government to respond to the crisis through the implementation of comprehensive HIV/AIDS programmes. The establishment of the Global Fund to Fight AIDS, Tuberculosis and Malaria (hereafter referred to as the Global Fund) in 2002 created a unique opportunity for the joint participation of public and private sector stakeholders in central issues of financing and implementing large-scale HIV/AIDS programmes and projects at country level. Soon after its establishment, the Global Fund signed a memorandum of understanding with the GBC to work together in promoting PPP in the HIV/AIDS response. This led to a particularly interesting application of PPP to HIV/AIDS response in the form of the 'co-investment' model, which is a mechanism to co-finance and support mutually beneficial joint HIV/AIDS service provision.

The co-investment model

The concept of co-investment has its origin in a joint working paper by the ILO and the Global Fund, prepared for a meeting in Evian, France, that was organised by private sector employers on the eve of the G8 Summit in July 2003 (ILO and GFATM 2003). The paper sought to clarify some of the basic principles and elaborate on practical elements for making use of PPPs to support the implementation of Global Fund grant projects at country level. It was intended to influence thinking about the role and contribution of the private sector to the newly established Global Fund, and co-investment was presented as a strategy for positioning the private sector to become a major partner of the Global Fund (Lavollay 2003).

The co-investment model has since been used by the Global Fund to encourage partnerships between the private sector and public sector authorities, and to promote the involvement of non-state actors in the planning and execution of Global Fund-financed HIV/AIDS projects at the country level (Cohen 2006; ILO/AIDS 2006). In addition to the Global Fund, the co-investment model has been applied to technical cooperation activities by the ILO, UNDP and WHO, and has also attracted the interest of major international and bilateral development agencies such as the World Bank, GTZ, the World Economic Forum, the Department for International Development (DFID), the Dutch Development Cooperation Programme and USAID (GBC 2004; Beckmann *et al.* 2005). The co-investment model has been endorsed and recommended by the GBC to its affiliates and membership worldwide, and this has led to the adoption of the model for HIV/AIDS response by well-known companies such as Unilever Tea in Kenya and Tanzania, Lafarge Cement in Nigeria, Daimler Chrysler in South Africa, Anglo American Group in South Africa, Ghana and Zimbabwe, Standard Chartered Bank in the Gambia and General Motors in Kenya (GBC 2003; 2004).

The co-investment model is recognised by the Global Fund as one of the options for involving representatives of business in the preparation and implementation of grant proposals submitted to the Fund by low- and middle-income countries. The model is seen as particularly relevant to the operation of the 'Country Coordinating Mechanism' (CCM)[3], which is the arrangement put in place by the Global Fund to ensure the participation of a wide range of stakeholders in the preparation and implementation of grant proposals submitted to the Fund. The thinking is that, by being a part of the CCM, business could influence grant proposals to include private sector participation in, and co-financing of, comprehensive and large-scale HIV/AIDS projects beyond the workplace on the basis of partnership with the public sector and other stakeholders. With this approach, it should be possible for the private sector to contribute additional resources for the implementation of HIV/AIDS projects that are financed primarily by the Global Fund and managed locally by public sector authorities.

The willingness of the private sector to contribute in this manner to national efforts to combat HIV/AIDS has been welcomed by the Global Fund as an ideal arrangement for involving the business in the Fund's processes. Hence, it was with tremendous excitement that the Global Fund announced in October 2003 that the Anglo American group in South Africa (a GBC member) had embarked on a ground-breaking co-investment scheme with the Fund and other partners, including the Nelson Mandela Foundation and the Henry J. Kaiser Foundation, to support a youth-oriented HIV/AIDS initiative, 'Love Life.' Anglo American's contribution to this initiative was the first example of how a private company can use the opportunities created by Global Fund financing to benefit the community at large through co-investment schemes (Global Fund 2004).

By 2004, a number of GBC-affiliated companies and national business coalitions had partnered with other stakeholders to prepare proposals on co-investment schemes for submission to the Global Fund. This was the case in Botswana, Ghana, Namibia, Zimbabwe and India, all of which submitted grant proposals to the Global Fund in 2005 and 2006 that incorporated components from private employers along the lines of co-investment schemes. The opportunities for corporate co-investment in Global Fund projects were not only limited to the proposal development phase, but extended to the participation of the private sector in subsequent phases of the Fund's project cycle (i.e. the grant negotiation, grant implementation and grant governance phases). This was indeed the case in Malawi, Tanzania, Uganda and the Gambia, where the private sector was involved in co-investment schemes at the grant implementation and governance phases (Global Fund 2004).

Well-known international companies, such as Anglo-American, Anglo Gold, BMW, Daimler Chrysler, General Motors, Lafarge, Heineken, Unilever, Chevron Texaco, Shell, Pfizer and Standard Chartered Bank have all made use of corporate co-investment schemes to partner with public sector authorities and NGOs in contributing to HIV/AIDS efforts at national and local level. Under co-investment schemes, the private sector has been involved in the preparation and execution of project proposals covering a variety of HIV/AIDS services, ranging from the establishment of voluntary counselling and testing (VCT) services, upgrading and expansion of community health facilities and home-based care, to training and capacity-building of the healthcare sector, procurement of drugs and leveraging of additional financial resources. The willingness of business to contribute to the wider national HIV/AIDS response, combined with the support provided by the government for co-investment schemes, attest to the efficacy of the private sector's role from both a governance and a business perspective.

The Global Fund particularly valued the opportunity provided by co-investment for private sector enterprises to put their healthcare infrastructure, including hospitals, clinics, drug procurement services and management experience into wider use as a public good for the benefit of the community. The former Executive Director of the Global Fund, Richard Feachem, summed up the advantage of this type of partnership as follows:

> 'Co-investment allows the private sector to contribute real assets and expertise to what must be a unique joint public/private collaboration in local communities (and) the Global Fund looks forward to providing financial support for this approach'
>
> (Global Fund 2004)

The importance of the availability of the private sector's health facilities for use by the local community is underlined by the fact that infrastructure costs have accounted for almost 40 per cent of the financial resources needed on average to scale up national HIV/AIDS programmes in countries such as Botswana, Kenya and Zambia (Lisk 2006a).

Partnership has been used by multinational and other large enterprises as the mechanism to extend the reach of workplace programmes to suppliers, contractors and local franchisees. In 2003, the Coca-Cola Company announced that all 40 Coca-Cola bottlers in Africa, which employ some 60,000 workers in 53 countries, have enrolled in the Coca-Cola Africa Foundation healthcare initiative to extend healthcare benefits to its independent bottlers in the region. The programme was intended to enable Coca-Cola's African bottlers to offer comprehensive HIV/AIDS awareness, prevention and care to their employees, their spouses and children. The Foundation was supposed to cover 50 per cent of the cost of the HIV/AIDS services, while the bottlers and employees would contribute 40 per cent and 10 per cent respectively. Implementation is decentralised, with each bottling company responsible for rolling out the programme at the local level.

Governance implications

Participation

The involvement of the private sector in the provision of treatment and care beyond the workplace allows for the wider community to benefit from those healthcare services, as some employers even go beyond the confines of HIV/AIDS services to address general community health needs. In some instances, the opening up of a private sector enterprise's healthcare facilities to the local community represents the first time that women have direct access to any type of healthcare. The extension of workplace HIV/AIDS programmes to the local community also provides a basis for workers and local people to participate in and benefit from the planning and execution of community health services. From a wider community development perspective, these extended workplace programmes usually relied on internal and external healthcare providers to create linkages with community health services; in some cases they led to community outreach initiatives in related areas such as training of community health workers, nutritionists and counsellors, and support for women involved in provision of homecare treatment, maternal care and childcare. It is important that representatives of workers and the community are involved right from the start in the organisation and, more crucially, the implementation and monitoring processes of these programmes. Another critical element is the multi-stakeholder approach to workplace strategy, which is manifested in the representation of management, trade unions and staff, and community organisations representing women, youth and migrant workers in the organisational structure of extended workplace programmes. This would ensure that the programmes address cultural sensitivities within the local context, promote communication and understanding between the different stakeholders, and foster a solid partnership that is based on mutual trust and therefore the sustainability of such programmes.

Poverty reduction, development impact and equity considerations

Implicit in the responsibility taken on by the private sector to address the wider development challenges of HIV/AIDS is a commitment to satisfy the health and other basic needs of workers and the community. The private sector has come to recognize the link between HIV/AIDS and poverty in many developing countries, and some firms have taken this into account in the formulation and implementation of HIV/AIDS workplace strategies and programmes. HIV/AIDS is a manifestation of existing poverty conditions that are partly the outcome of insufficient incomes and unsustainable livelihoods and partly the result of the impact of the epidemic on socioeconomic conditions. Consequently, the maintenance and expansion of poverty through the spread of HIV/AIDS harms the community and holds back development, which is also not good for business. Conversely, reduction in poverty through improved response to and governance of HIV/AIDS in the community is good for development and business.

Policy and programme responses to HIV/AIDS by the private sector could reduce the economic and social costs of the epidemic to business and also contribute overall to efforts to reduce poverty and promote a more equitable and sustainable pattern of development. Just how private sector interventions can contribute to improved governance, in terms of poverty reduction and equity, requires an understanding of the relationship between income and health. As a major employer of labour, the private sector has a vested interest in important human resource indicators such as labour productivity, education and skill levels. A healthy and educated workforce is an important factor in sustaining enterprises and keeping them profitable. The most important contribution of the private sector's HIV/AIDS interventions to poverty reduction and equity is perhaps through the impact of such interventions on human capital. The deprivation of human capital is itself a form of poverty, which is linked to the governance of the AIDS epidemic in terms of the loss of capacity to develop and utilise human capabilities to respond to the epidemic. Interventions in the private sector that reduce the risk to HIV infection and prolong working life are critical to reducing poverty at all levels.

Extending HIV/AIDS workplace programmes to the local community constitutes a basis for improvements in the health status of the community, which could improve access to income-generating opportunities and enhance livelihoods. This in turn could help to reduce poverty and inequality. The additional contribution of the private sector should reduce the economic and social costs to the government of responding to HIV/AIDS, and leave the public sector with greater fiscal space to address poverty. Furthermore, it is likely that improvement in the health status of the general population would be more beneficial to the poor disproportionately, which as a socioeconomic group depends more on physical labour as a productive asset for earning an income than other groups. Empowerment of the poor – which includes women who are usually disadvantaged because of societal biases and discriminatory practices based on cultural and traditional norms – through improved access to healthcare, employment and other socioeconomic opportunities has significant equity and governance implications.

High risk groups and gender dimensions

HIV/AIDS affects the most impoverished, marginalised and disadvantaged groups in the population. Women, children and youth, migrant and mobile workers, sex workers and people working in the informal economy are at particular risk (Cohen 1998; 2006; Lisk 2002). The reasons for their vulnerability are well documented in ILO and other publications (ILO 2002; Lisk 2006b; Hodges 2004; UNAIDS 2008). The important point to emphasise is that workplace programmes and practices in HIV/AIDS care and support have been successful in developing interventions that target these groups as part of their response to the impact of the epidemic in the private sector. For example, Anglo American mines in South Africa have supported alternative income-generation programmes for women whose husband have been retrenched due to AIDS-related illness, while Daimler Chrysler South Africa has included special education and information activities for men aimed at changing sexual behaviour in its HIV/AIDS prevention programmes and 'How to be a responsible man' campaigns (GBC 2001; GBC website resources). In India, the Tata Iron and Steel Company's workplace HIV/AIDS programme includes the formation of a 'Ladies Core Group' which focuses on education and awareness-raising targeted at women who are unable to address their problems due to social inhibition (GBC, resources). In recognising the wider causes of the spread of HIV in terms of the sexual behaviour of their large male immigrant worker population, especially with respect to commercial sex workers, mining companies in South Africa have entered into multi-sectoral partnerships with local NGOs to implement projects that provide medical assistance and counselling for sex workers and women of limited economic resources who enter into sexual relationship with miners for money or material support (UNAIDS/GBC/PWBLF 2000). Old Mutual Insurance and Financial Services, a South African company, supports a number of independently run HIV/ADS orphans programmes across the country for children who have lost their parents to the epidemic, and encourages its staff to 'adopt an orphan', whereby employees make monthly contributions from their salaries towards financially supporting one or more orphans (GHI/WEF 2006; WEF-GHI website resources).

Conclusion: Lessons, policy interventions and practical action-oriented results

The private sector has become increasingly involved in the fight against HIV/AIDS, not only for reasons of business interest but also for humanitarian reasons linked to a sense of CSR. Concern by firms about the impact of the epidemic on productivity and profitability, as well as the effect on their corporate image, underpin a strategy in which the private sector takes responsibility for the governance and delivery of HIV/AIDS services. The private sector in many instances has qualities and facilities, problem-solving expertise and entrepreneurial spirit, which can be decisive in AIDS response. Partnerships with the public sector and other stakeholders at national and local levels have been useful in extending the reach of private sector HIV/AIDS interventions beyond the workplace, indicating the potential of the private sector to contribute to an effective HIV/AIDS response and mitigate the wider development impacts of the epidemic across communities.

Reaching out to communities is vital to the effectiveness of workplace HIV/AIDS programmes offered by the private sector. The community, as emphasised in the ILO Code of Practice, is where firms get their workers from and should be regarded as an extension of the workplace. Furthermore, the community is where people's attitudes and behaviours are formed, reinforced and changed. By reaching into their communities, workplaces can be instrumental in helping to remove societal barriers and obstacles that fuel the transmission of HIV and keep women and other vulnerable groups at high risk to infection. Investments by private sector enterprises in community-level programmes also generate capacity, and mobilise resources and people to respond effectively to HIV/AIDS.

The Political Declaration on HIV/AIDS adopted by the UN General Assembly in June 2006 recognises the important role of the private sector in HIV prevention and care, and in the treatment of AIDS. Direct business action will ensure benefits that maintain efficiency and productivity of enterprise operations, as well as protect their greatest resource – human capital. Experience and lessons learned so far suggest that the private sector in many highly affected countries, on account of its resources and experience, will continue to influence national capacity to respond effectively to HIV/AIDS as a development challenge. The resources and vibrancy of the private sector could help to surmount existing barriers in the fight against HIV/AIDS and improve the reach of current efforts. The participation of the private sector as a major stakeholder in the HIV/AIDS response should therefore be encouraged and promoted in public policy, both for meeting the need for an effective response to the epidemic and for improving the governance of the response.

Notes

1 The ILO is an international organisation within the UN system that has a tripartite structure, made up of representatives of governments, employers' and workers' organisations from over 190 member states.

2 The Millennium Development Goals (MDGs) are time-bound targets established by the UN to halve extreme poverty globally by 2015; one of the 8 MDGs ia aimed at controlling and reversing the spread of HIV by 2015. There is a widespread belief within the UN and among members of the international community that the impact of HIV/AIDS could jeopardise the achievement of the other MDGs in many developing countries.

3 The Country Coordinating Mechanism (CCM) was set up as an essential structure of the Global Fund's architecture and underlined its commitment to local ownership and broad-based participation of all major stakeholders, including non-state actors, in the decision-making process. The typical CCM includes as such representatives from both the public and private sectors, as well as multilateral and bilateral development agencies, NGOs and civil society organisations, as well as associations of PLWHA, and is charged with the responsibility to develop and

submit grant proposals to the Global Fund, based on priority needs at the national level. After grant approval, the CCM is also responsible for overseeing and monitoring progress during implementation of the proposal.

Bibliography

Barnett, T. and Whiteside, A. (2002). *AIDS in the twenty-first century: Disease and globalization*. Basingstoke: Palgrave Macmillan.

Beckmann, S., Rai, P., Alli, B.O., Lisk, F., Mulanga, C., Lavollay, M. and Girrbach, E. (2005). *HIV/AIDS workplace programmes and Public-Private-Partnerships through Co-investment – Extension of Treatment and Care into the Community*, Geneva: ILO.

Bonnel, R. (2000). 'HIV/AIDS and economic growth: A global perspective', *The South African Journal of Economics*, (68)5: 820–54.

Cohen, D. (1998). 'The HIV epidemic and sustainable human development', *Issues Paper No. 29*, New York: UNDP.

—— (2002). 'Human Capital and HIV/AIDS epidemic in Sub-Saharan Africa', *Working Paper No. 2, ILO Programme on HIV/AIDS and the World of Work (ILO/AIDS)*. Geneva.

Cohen, D. (2006). 'Responding to the challenges of poverty and HIV/AIDS in Zambia', *Paper prepared for Zambia National AIDS Council Stakeholders Meeting, 27–29 January, Lusaka,* UNDP.

Greener, R. (1997). 'Impact of HIV/AIDS and options for intervention; Results of a five-company pilot study'. *Working Paper 10, Botswana Institute of Development Policy Analysi.,* Gaberone.

Global Business Coalition on HIV/AIDS (GBC) (2001). *Business action on HIV/AIDS–A blueprint*. New York.

GBC (2003). 'Nine Major Companies Commit to Co-investment to Expand Community HIV/AIDS Programs using Corporate Infrastructure', Press Release, Nairobi, December 3, 2003.

—— (2004). *Co-investment: A mechanism for engaging businesses in the fight against HIV/AIDS*, New York.

—— Resources: Managing HIV in the workplace (http://www.gbcaids.com/wpp_tools.asp)

Global Fund to Fight AIDS, Tuberculosis and Malaria (GFATM) (2004). *Co-investment scheme at country level*. Geneva.

Global Health Initiative (GHI)/ World Economic Forum (WEF) (2006). *Annual global business survey, 2005–2006*, Geneva

GHI/WEF (2008). *Business coalitions tackling AIDS: A worldwide review, January 2008*. Geneva

Hacker, M. (2001). *The economic consequences of HIV/AIDS in Southern Africa*, IMF, Washington DC.

Hodges, J. (2004). 'Guidelines for addressing HIV/AIDS in the workplace through employment and labour law', *Working Paper No.3, ILO-IFP/DIALOGUE*, Geneva.

ILO (2000). *Implementing the ILO Code of Practice on HIV/AIDS and the World of Work: An education and training manual*. Geneva

——(2001). *An ILO code of practice on HIV/AIDS and the world of work*. Geneva.

——(2003). 'The ILO perspective on the integrated approach to occupational safety and health', *Working Document, 13th Session of ILO/WHO Committee on Occupational Health*, 9–12 December. Geneva.

—— (2004). *Global strategy on occupational safety and health.* Conclusions adopted by the International Labour Conference at its 91st Session 2003. Geneva.

ILO and GFATM (2003). *Co-investment: A central mechanism for establishing PPP at country level*, Geneva: ILO.

ILO Programme on HIV/AIDS and the World of Work (2006). *HIV/AIDS and Work in a Globalizing World.* Geneva: ILO.

——(2004). *HIV/AIDS and Work: Global Estimates, Impact and Response*, Geneva: ILO.

ILO/AIDS

International Finance Corporation (IFC) (2002). Good practice note: HIV/AIDS in the workplace. Washington.

Lavollay, M. (2003). *The Global Fund – Co-investment schemes at country level.* Geneva: ILO.

Lisk, F. (2002). 'The Labour Market and Employment Implications of HIV/AIDS', *Working Paper, No.1*, ILO/AIDS, Geneva.

—— (2006a). 'The Co-investment Model: A Public Private Partnership Strategy for improving access to HIV/AIDS services'. *Paper presented at the International Conference on HIV/AIDS and Business: Challenges for Sustainable Development, Westminster University Business School*, London, 7–8 September.

—— (2006b). 'Development and Human Rights implications of HIV/AIDS: Issues and challenges.' *Paper presented at Annual Conference of the Norwegian Association for Development Research*, Oslo, 13–15 September.

—— (2006c). 'AIDS and governance: The development dimension', *UNDP Background Pape.* New York.

—— (2008) 'Towards a New Architecture of Global Governance for Responding to the HIV/AIDS Epidemic' in Cooper,A, Hocking,B and Maley,W (eds) (2008), *Global governance and diplomacy: Worlds Apart?* Basingstoke: Palgrave Macmillan.

Lisk, F. and Cohen, D. (2007). 'Regional responses to HIV/AIDS: A Global Public Goods Approach' in Poku, N., Whiteside, A. and Sandkjaer, B. (eds), *AIDS and Governance.* Aldershot: Ashgate.

McPherson, M.F. (2002). 'HIV/AIDS, human capacity and institutions: Sustaining economic growth'. *Paper prepared for USAID Biennial Conference on strategies for responding to HIV/AIDS*, Washington DC, February.

McPherson, M.F, in association with Hoover, D. and Snodgrass, D. (2000). 'The impact of economic growth in Africa of rising costs and labour productivity losses associated with HIV/AIDS'. *Paper prepared for the CAER-II project, Kennedy School of Government*, Harvard University, August.

Natrass, N., Neilson, T., Bery, P., Mistry, N. and Sievers, S.E. (2005). ' Opportunities for Business in the fight against HIV/AIDS', *GBC Discussion Paper.* New York.

Over, M. (1992). 'The macroeconomic impact of AIDS in Sub-Saharan Africa' *AFTPN Technical Working Paper No.3,* Washington, DC: World Bank.

Organization of African Unity (OAU) (2001). 'Abuja Declaration on HIV/AIDS, Tuberculosis and other related infectious diseases', *OAU Special Summit, Abuja, Nigeria*, April.

Piot, P. (2002). 'AIDS chain reaction threatens sustainable development'. *Address to the World Summit on Sustainable Development*, Johannesburg, August 30, UNAIDS Press Release: Geneva.

Ramachandran, V, Manju, K. and Turner, G. (2006). 'Does the private sector care about AIDS? Evidence from investment climate surveys in East Africa' *Working Paper No. 76, Centre for Global Development, January 2006.* Washington DC.

Roderick, A. (2004). 'Governance and AIDS in West Africa', *Justice Africa*

Rosen, S., Simon J., Vincent, J., MacLeod, W., Fox, M.,and Thea, D.M. (2003). 'AIDS is your business', *Harvard Business Review*, February 2003, pp. 81–87.

Sachs, J. (2005). *Investing in development: A practical plan to achieve the Millennium Development Goals.* New York: UN Millennium Project.

United Nations (UN) (1979). 'Convention on the elimination of all forms of discrimination against women' (CEDAW), *General Assembly Resolution 34/180.* New York.

UN (2000). 'Millennium Development Declaration', *United Nations General Assembly Millennium Development Summit*, September 2000. New York.

—— (2001). 'Declaration of commitment on HIV/AIDS', *United Nations General Assembly Special Session on HIVAIDS (UNGASS) Resolution S26–2*, New York, 25–27 June.

—— (2006). 'Political Declaration on HIV/AIDS' *UN General Assembly,* New York.

United Nations Development Programme (UNDP) (2007). *Governance and HIV/AIDS responses: Issues and outlook.* New York

United Nations Joint Programme on HIV/AIDS (UNAIDS) (1998). *Gender and HIV/AIDS.* Geneva.

—— (2001). Top businesses pledge to act on HIV/AIDS, GBC-UNAIDS Press Release, New York, 26 June.

—— (2002). The private sector responds to the epidemic: Debswana – a global benchmark. Geneva.

—— (2005). *Access to treatment in the private-sector workplace.* A joint publication with ILO, WHO and GBC. Geneva

—— (2008). *Report on the global AIDS epidemic.* Geneva

UNAIDS/GBC/The Prince of Wales Business Leaders Forum (PWBLF) (2000). *The business response to HIV/AIDS: The impact of lessons learned.* Geneva and London.

UNAIDS and World Health Organisation (WHO) (2007). *AIDS Epidemic Update: December 2000.* Geneva.

UNDP/Government of Malawi (2002). *The impact of HIV/AIDS on human resources in Malawi.* Lilongwe, Malawi: UNDP.

Vass, J. (2005). *The impact of HIV/AIDS on the labour market in South Africa,* Human Sciences Research Council. Cape Town, South Africa.

Whiteside, A. (2008). *HIV/AIDS: A very short introduction.* Oxford: Oxford University Press.

World Bank (2000). *Intensifying Action against HIV/AIDS in Africa: Responding to Development Crisis.* Washington DC.

World Economic Forum (WEF) (2004). *Business and HIV/AIDS: Who me? A global review of the business response to HIV/AIDS 2003–2004.* Geneva.

WEF-GHI: Private sector intervention case example: Old Mutual (http://www.weforum.org/globalhealth)

World Health Assembly (2006). 'Women, children and AIDS', *WHA 43.10.* Geneva: WHO.

World Health Organisation (WHO) (2004). *Investing in a comprehensive health response sector to HIV/AIDS.* Geneva.

Part IV

Global Governance and Multisectoralism

7 Institutional participation, accountability and transparency in the HIV/AIDS response

A case for Zimbabwe

Felicity Hatendi-Gutu

This chapter does not directly assess Zimbabwe's governance performance; rather the objective of the chapter is to contribute to the strengthening of country-level institutional dimensions of governance within the HIV/AIDS response, through the sharing of in-country experiences. This is in relation to key administrative structures and processes linked to the multisectoral HIV/AIDS response in Zimbabwe. The premise is that reports and communication must be made in the context that society, donors and other development partners now demand transparency and greater accountability from recipients of resources. This is with particular reference to institutions involved in the good governance undertaking and the management of the localised HIV/AIDS response, with particular regards to their financial and non-financial affairs.[1] Transparency in the allocation of funds and programme actions are essential to gain the widespread support from all stakeholders involved in addressing the HIV/AIDS looming funding crisis (Akukwe 2005).[2] The heightened call for organisational accountability and transparency suggests that not all organisations and structures involved in HIV/AIDS are accountable or transparent, or adhere to good governance criteria or practices. In fact, it is commonly perceived that some governance structures lack credibility within society and amongst funding agencies. In agreement, Poku *et al.* suggest that generally in Africa, key in-country institutions have been affected by a history of poor governance and with the effects of high HIV/AIDS prevalence rates, resulting in weakened public sectors, and as such institutions cannot really be expected to be functional (Poku *et al.*. 2007).

This chapter focuses on institutional governance. It begins by describing the operational context of HIV/AIDS in Zimbabwe and the resources involved with the multisectoral response. Within the description of the in-country institutional governance structures, particular attention is given to the National AIDS Council (NAC)-administered National AIDS Trust Fund (NATF) as a key local funding institution and the Global Fund to Fight AIDS, Tuberculosis and Malaria (hereafter Global Fund). Discussions will acknowledge the five dimensions articulated by the South African Development Community (SADC) that underpin good governance and equally sustainable development, namely political, institutional, economic, social and gender (SADC 2000). Reference is made to the administrative structures and processes through which HIV/AIDS policy design, implementation, monitoring and evaluation occur, and the institutional governance challenges faced by the local institutions (Strode and Grant 2004). In conclusion, it will be argued that in an increasingly resource-constrained environment, key administrative institutions, structures and processes need to be inclusive rather than exclusive in their recognition, undertaking and compliance of the core norms of good governance. These include participation[3] transparency,[4] responsiveness,[5] consensus-building, effectiveness and efficiency and accountability[6] with regard to the provision of HIV/AIDS services and goods. Accountable organisations should respond to the following basic, commonly asked questions: *What* is being accounted for? To *Whom*? and *How*? The paper draws on information gathered from the United Nations Development Programme (UNDP) position papers, in-country Global Fund administrative structures, NAC and Global Fund discussion papers, Global Fund grant recipients' progress reports and review meetings. For the purposes of this paper 'stakeholders' will refer to internal (national) stakeholders unless otherwise specified. An internal organisational stakeholder refers to individuals and groups that can be infected and or are affected by the organisation's policies and are a formal part of the organization. External stakeholders are not formally part of the organisation but can be affected by organisational decisions.

Background and context

With a population of 11.6 million, Zimbabwe continues to have one of the highest HIV/AIDS prevalence rates in the world (CSO 2002). It was estimated that by the end of 2005, the country had 1.61 million people living with HIV (Zimbabwe national estimate of HIV, 2005); there was a noted decline in 2007, with a prevalence of 15.6 per cent in comparison to 18 per cent in 2006 (Zimbabwe Demographic Health Survey 2005–6; UNAIDS 2005). Despite the significant government commitment to the multisectoral response to HIV/AIDS in Zimbabwe, however, the epidemic remains problematic. The number of people dying of AIDS-related diseases during 2007 was estimated at 115,114, bringing the number of living HIV/AIDS orphans to 975,956 (Zimbabwe national estimate of HIV, 2007). The estimated number of adults (age 15–49) needing universal access to antiretroviral drugs (ARVs) peaked at 510.356 in 2004 and was 479, 796 in 2007 with approximately 86,000 people receiving ARVs at that time through the 2004 national rollout exercise. Demand continues to outstrip supply. The attainment of Millennium Development Goal 6 remains a challenge under the current economic environment.[7] The HIV/AIDS situation is compounded by an increasingly hyperinflationary environment of around 14,000 per cent in 2007 (CSO 2007). Declining economic performance, high unemployment, and shortages in fuel, food, drugs and foreign currency, a decline in donor funding, and political tensions, remain areas of concern, and have resulted in increased levels of poverty. The country faces declining health services provision as a result of factors such as the brain drain, ageing equipment and infrastructure, shortages of basic drugs, the collapse of a once-excellent referral system and health services that are inaccessable and unaffordable for the majority of people (UNGASS 2006).

Zimbabwe receives its financial allocations for HIV/AIDS from three main sources namely the: national budget allocation, the NATF, commonly referred to as the HIV/AIDS levy, and long-term loans from donors. The people's access to services and resources is largely determined by government policies. Other funds are received through independent budgets that do not contribute to the national budget directly. Different methods are commonly used for financial accounting and reporting and the Zimbabwe National HIV and AIDS Strategic Plan (ZNASP, 2007) refers to the need for standardisation and harmonisation of systems, including the need for gender-disaggregated reporting, and minimal discrepancies in financial and non-financial data collection. As Transparency International Zimbabwe cited in 2007, donor funds and government budget allocations for combatting HIV/AIDS seem to have presented both an enormous opportunity and a great temptation, as there are growing allegations of misuse of these funds by the institutions and individuals administering them.

Zimbabwe remains one of the many African countries yet to realise the terms of the Abuja Declaration on HIV/AIDS, Tuberculosis and Other Related Infectious Diseases of 2000, in which African leaders pledged to allocate 15 per cent of their national budgets to healthcare. It has been noted that the total domestic spending by people and governments accounts for a significant part of the local, national and global response. It is generally argued that domestic spending on HIV/AIDS usually increases as the national budget increases as a result of improvement in trade, greater productivity, or debt relief. This has not been the case in Zimbabwe as a result of the stagnation of its economy over the past years. Analysis of the national budget allocation to the Zimbabwean healthcare sector overall has shown a declining trend. For example, the Ministry of Health and Child Welfare in 2007 allocated 1.2 trillion Zimbabwean dollars to health; this was against an inflation rate of 20,000 per cent. This allocation was expected to procure health services and supplies such as the much-needed ARVs in foreign currency amid a national foreign currency shortage. As a result of the hyperinflationary environment, insufficient amounts of ARVs were eventually procured and the government struggled with, and eventually failed to meet, its own coverage target by the end of 2007.

Faced with declining foreign aid and bilateral donations, the Zimbabwe government responded to repeat domestic calls to mobilise and prioritise its own resources for the national response to the epidemic. This worked despite the governance challenges faced by the country's diminished input from external sources. The NATF – the first of its kind in Africa – was set up to ease Zimbabwe's reliance on external funding in the HIV/AIDS response and was established in terms of Section 30 of the Audit and Exchequer Act (MoF 1999) in 1999. The overall objective of the NATF remains to mobilise and provide local funding for the realisation of the objectives of the 1999 National AIDS policy, National HIV/AIDS Strategic Framework (NSF) 2000–2004, together with the recently adopted and revised Zimbabwe National HIV/AIDS Strategic Plan (ZNASP) 2006–2010. The NATF contributions form a large and important part of the national contribution to the multisectoral national AIDS response.

The Permanent Secretary of the Ministry of Health and Child Welfare provides an oversight role whilst the Zimbabwe NAC Board administers the fund using existing governance tools and instruments.[8] All administrative and accounting procedures are undertaken in accordance with NATF policies and guidelines. The Trust funds are made up of a 3 per cent individual monthly AIDS levy taxed from those gainfully employed in the formal sector and through corporate taxes. The total amount of financial resources that flow into the NATF on a monthly and annual basis is not disclosed to the public. Fund expenditures relate to existing cases of HIV/AIDS and new national programmes in the following priority areas: prevention, treatment, care, mitigation and research. These are complemented by donor support from the Global Fund. Expanded expenditures include core expenditures as well as health care expenses such as health facility-based care and treatment. Funds are disbursed through decentralised NAC structures and approved annual plans that are responsive to defined community needs and priorities, on a phased basis. Selective capacity building is undertaken to support NAC decentralised structures and enhance their financial management, documentation, and activity-reporting abilities. Reports are channeled to the NAC and the responsible line ministry. Decentralisation increases transparency, and the amount of money that can be diverted from development programmes often declines in countries that pursue this approach (UNDP 2003).

The objective of decentralisation, and importantly fiscal decentralisation, is to bring decision making closer to the people and enhance levels of participation. This has generally not been the answer for ensuring delivery of HIV/AIDS services at the grassroots level, as not all local district, ward and village authorities have enough power to make collective budget decisions – due to skills, capacity and resource shortages. This compromises efficient and effective resource management and the responsiveness of the localised HIV/AIDS response, as the voices of the most needy including women and children remain marginalised. The need to reform institutional structures in Africa to enhance efficiency, effectiveness and governance practices in service delivery, and to reduce the likelihood of corruption is obvious to decision-makers and implementers at all levels. What is generally lacking is the means to sustain enforcement of policies that could lead to meaningful change in resource allocation and distribution.[9] That there are problems relating to institutional capacities and mechanisms to ensure effectiveness, transparency and accountability in Sub-Saharan Africa is generally accepted, although the severity of these problems is said to vary from country to country. Shortfalls in institutional capacity in the areas of policy-making and implementation have been cited in Zimbabwe (Agere 1998).

In a continuing effort to address governance deficits, the recipients of the NATF funds are required to meet stipulated institutional capacity intervention criteria and address issues relating to project sustainability requirements. These include: (i) the evidence of: adequate institutional human resources and capacities; (ii) the presence of functional accounting and reporting, monitoring and evaluation systems and processes; (iii) relevant HIV/AIDS programming experiences; and (iv) a well-grounded understanding of the local dynamics and impact of the epidemic. Civil society organisations (CSOs) as key non-state NATF grant recipients have made attempts to enhance these values through the development and adoption of the Zimbabwe NGO Code of Ethics. Though policing remains weak, it is a step in the right direction. The NATF faces increased funding demands as result of dwindling national and donor resources to combat HIV/AIDS in Zimbabwe, with service demands outstripping supply. Weakened local recipients with lowered absorptive capacities have highlighted the need to address emerging governance issues relating to transparency, participation and accountability.

Good governance emphasises the full participation of all parties, and the presence of functional institutional processes and structures that enable all stakeholders to play an active role in decision-making processes and activities that affect them. The full participation of all requires HIV/AIDS programmes to be people-centred and gender-sensitive, which in turn will increase the programme's level of responsiveness to people's needs, particularly the needs of poor and marginalised groups. This requires additional local skills and capacities to be developed in order to attain this goal. The current NAC Board and the NAC decentralised structures are highly representative in their composition – members are drawn from the public, private and civil society sectors, including labour unions, ordinary men, women and young people (NAC 2001). The particular role and significant contribution of people living with HIV/AIDS (PLWHAs), young people, women and CSOs in addressing the problem of HIV/AIDS in the design, planning, implementation and evaluation of programmes is crucial to the development of effective responses to the HIV/AIDS epidemic (UN 2001). The NAC enhances accountability in line with 'The Three Ones' requirements of one national coordinating structure, one monitoring and evaluation system and one HIV/AIDS coordinating framework.[10] The decentralised NAC structures undertake the coordination of the national HIV/AIDS response, which involves financial and programmatic monitoring and evaluation.

The members of the NAC are responsible and accountable to varied constituents. Representatives possess different levels of education, awareness and empowerment, and thus the level of participation in these structures differ. Patronage systems have reportedly influenced the degree of meaningful participation within the decentralised structures to a small degree. As mechanisms are not in place in the NATF and the decentralised NAC institutions for the effective participation of all, this has often resulted in limited opportunities to place questions on the HIV/AIDS agenda, and reduced the ability to express individual and community preferences as to the outcome of decision-making within these implementing bodies. Lack of information plays a key part in weak participation levels as people often lack access to data that is in the hands of officials. This may be attributed to the failure by officials in the decentralised structures to produce and disseminate relevant, appropriate and updated HIV/AIDS and NATF information. Efforts are in place to enhance direct or indirect participation through informed representation of the people's views and opinions, as reported by elected or nominated leaders within the central and decentralised structures of the NAC, such as provincial and district committees. Measures to ensure this require the representatives to be located at the grassroots, living with the infected and affected persons and communities. The participation levels of women, young people, rural and remote populations, the disabled, and other vulnerable groups in local governance remains marginal, with the need for improved appropriate and timely HIV/AIDS communication and information. Evidence suggests that Zimbabwe has done little to narrow gender inequality according to the 2007 World Economic Forum report. The Gender Index of the same year ranks Zimbabwe 88th out of 128 surveyed countries.

NGOs in the multi-level and multisectoral response are members of the decentralised committees such as District Action Committees (DACs) and continue to undertake activities and programmes that complement those of government. Although they are sometimes regarded as running diametric activities due to the limited interaction, information exchange, communication, and planning with state structures, members of the decentralised NAC structures suggest that this is because they often lack awareness of the national guidelines and clarity on their roles and responsibilities in the multisectoral response. By and large, they play a vital role in the delivery of HIV/AIDS services to the local community levels in the absence of government decentralised structures reaching the grassroots level. A further strength of NGOs in the current environment is their ability to raise much-needed external funds. However, NGOs continue to point out that they have little scope to influence the national agenda within the specific parameters that are unilaterally set by the donor organisations who remain the biggest funders of their HIV/AIDS development programmes. NGO accountability is diverse – the majority are directly accountable to their external funders for organisational operations in the field; a situation that has caused increasingly strained relations between the government and civil society. The use of internal management systems, reporting instruments and detailed written procedures of accountability has generally evolved within civil society as a result of donor pressure to test NGO accountability (Moyo *et al.* 2000). Further to enhance the level of CSO stakeholder social accountability with regards to resource management, the government introduced the Private Voluntary Organisation

(PVO) Act Chapter 17:05 2007. The Act ensures accountability and makes mandatory the need for CSOs to notify local authorities of their presence in the area. According to the Act, the CSOs should seek the consent and facilitation of respective line ministries in their operations and should be supervised by local authorities. The registering authority should monitor the CSO activities by undertaking field visits to project areas and ensure submission of annual narrative reports and audited financial statements.

Transparency in the use of the HIV/AIDS funds through the provision of accessible and timely information to stakeholders and opening up of organisational procedures, structures and processes to their assessment, still remains inaccessible to the majority of the people. Transparency involves broad participatory and transparent information and communication within an open political culture. In such a culture, all media and communication services are generally treated as public and benevolent. In a study in Uganda, Byanyima discussed how government officials were often reluctant to share government information, but after working with NGOs and understanding their roles and contribution, they became convinced of the value of their work and began to facilitate access to government documentation, overcoming a long tradition of official secrecy (Byanyima 2000). At times, information circulating in the decentralised structures of the NAC has allowed local stakeholders and other interested parties to report and act on the possible abuse of resources in defence of the public interests. There was a lot of controversy surrounding the NATF disbursements made in 2002 to the Zimbabwe National Association of Positive People in the Auditor General's report. Media reports alleged misuse and abuse of funds and resources allocated to the organisation. Hence in a bid to enhance public information surrounding the NATF operations, the NAC published the NATF beneficiary institutions, a practice that it has since stopped, with the NAC citing resource constraints.

The NAC structures embarked on the participatory development of HIV/AIDS plans, seeking to incorporate the views from the grassroot levels. The composition of the national, provincial, district, ward and village level committees also reflect the attempts to have the voices of the vulnerable groups heard at the various decision- and policy-making levels through their broad-based representation. However, it is evident that there is a need for recognition of the needs and potential of these groups in order to represent the interests of vulnerable groups. In order to make meaningful contributions, it is essential for representatives to have a sufficient grasp of technical and professional issues that is based on a firm understanding of the structures and procedures in place. The common challenges are the lack of specialised planning and technical skills on the part of group members and the intended direct beneficiaries. All efforts to improve the level of governance within the NAC and its administration of the NATF are geared to address public concerns over governance issues such as transparency, accountability and commonly perceived bureaucratic tendencies, whilst raising the level of public discussion and debate on the NATF (NAC 2001).

Additional financial resources continue to be mobilised through multilateral, bilateral donors and partners that include the GFATM, United Nations Agencies, United States Agency for International Development (USAID), and the European Union, which scale treatment and prevention activities in Zimbabwe (WHO 2005). The European Union supports the Expanded Support Programme (ESP) and targets the initiation of 16,000 additional and existing 6,000 clients on ARVs in its first year of operations. This will augment the Global Fund Round One and Five grants bringing an estimated total figure of nearly 59, 000 clients on ARVs (The Standard Supplement World AIDS Day, 25th November 2007).

Global Fund HIV/AIDS resources for the multisectoral response

The Global Fund resources augment the existing NATF and national health budgetary allocation, as do dwindling conditional grants from external sources. The resources contribute to the reduction of the spread of HIV in Zimbabwe, improvement of the quality of life of those infected and affected, and mitigation of the socioeconomic impact of the epidemic in Zimbabwe. The Global Fund turned down Zimbabwean proposals in five of seven funding rounds, but it continues to make significant financial contributions to the multisectoral response. Of the Round One, Phase One grant, a total of US $7,830,752.87 was disbursed over a two-year period and Round Five provided US$35.9 million in 2007. All grant funds were released following the meeting of conditions and focused on attempting to cut the exchange rate losses that were being encountered as a result of the hyperinflationary environment. Good governance practices are increasingly conditional to continued receipt of development assistance and foreign aid as the Zimbabwean economic decline continues.

The grant funds support the national implementation and scaling up of interventions, focusing on strengthening existing prevention of HIV among young people, provision of community home based care, scaling up of ARV treatment, expansion of Voluntary Counselling and Testing (VCT) services, prevention of mother-to-child transmission (PMTCT). Round Five grant funds will support the scaling-up of the existing ART programme. Those in-country institutions involved in the application, execution and management of the institutional governance norms within the Global Fund are namely the local fund agent (LFA), country coordinating mechanism (CCM), principal recipients, sub-recipients and sub-sub-recipients. These actors are directly or indirectly charged with the institutional governance of three Global Fund programme resources, namely financial, human and material resources. The Global Fund institutions work hand in hand with the state, respective line ministries, NAC structures and civil society. The inputs are translated into activities such as support to existing health services, delivery of income transfers, and rehabilitation of infrastructure. Outputs relate to numbers of Global Fund patients screened, tested, counselled and provided with ARVs, and young people receiving AIDS education. The Global Fund programmatic outcomes and impact indicators are in relation to the national programme, project and activities supported, and reporting on measures of progress, within the agreed-upon country-level monitoring and evaluation system. General access to this information, however, remains problematic: placing information in the public domain remains a challenge.

Global Fund institutional governance dimensions

These include all who have an interest and are directly or indirectly affected by the Global Fund operations and policies within the public (including government), private, civil society sectors, and their respective decentralised institutions, through to the communities and individuals infected and or affected by the HIV virus. The key Global Fund institutions – the LFA and principle recipients, etc. – allow for varying degrees of participation to ensure that their institutional processes allow internal stakeholders to play an active role in the decision-making processes and activities. The ordinary grassroots men and women, PLWHAs, and other marginalised groups face difficulties in engaging with these structures, and are commonly ignored. For example the LFA – whilst offering a wide range of audit and assurance transactions, crisis management, performance improvement, tax and human resource services, tailored to suit the industry or sector that it is offering these services to – allows for only minimal participation in the core elements of its Global Fund activity. The LFA is not considered a public institution, but rather the 'eyes and ears' and in-country representative of the Global Fund. Limited information about this important GFATM policy and decision-making body, and its roles and responsibilities led to varied perceptions of the LFA as a fully fledged CCM member, a spy, an observer, and/or a technical advisor.[11] The roles and responsibilities of the LFAs were later clarified in a Global Fund, Geneva letter to all principal recipients in the Southern African cluster of September 2006, which was circulated to relevant in-country stakeholders.

Contracted by the Global Fund, the LFA is duty-bound to provide grant financial management oversight, undertake grant negotiations, assess the principal recipient's capacity to implement the grant, review proposed budgets and work plans, and independently oversee programme performance and accountability in the use of funds (known as 'verification of implementation'). Other roles include reviewing the principal recipients' quarterly periodic requests for funds, the undertaking of site visits to verify programme results, and the reviewing of the principal recipients annual audit reports. All the services provided to the CCM and principal recipients are deemed crucial in assisting the Global Fund Geneva to make decisions on whether to continue funding beyond the initial two years of the grant cycle. Public participation, communication and dialogue are largely restricted to the Global Fund in Geneva, the CCM and principal recipients. The LFA's complaints and response mechanism addresses the concerns of in-country Global Fund stakeholders, with respect to organisational decisions and actions. However, the organisational processes that should ensure these complaints are properly reviewed remain unclear.

The role of the CCM, a representative and also a self-perpetuating board, is the coordination of national Global Fund proposals, selection of principal recipients, monitoring of grant implementation, and to approve major changes in the operational plans. It is constituted according to Global Fund Geneva guidelines,[12] and it has a mandate to perform evaluations of grant performance (oversight role), and ensure local strategic partnership building, linkages and consistency between the Global Fund assistance, and other health and development programmes in line with the national plans.[13] Whilst the CCM has several notable strengths, and exhibits a high degree of the Global Fund programme ownership, it has several shortcomings in the execution of its 'governance role'.[14] These include no direct links to the grassroots population, a limited oversight role and an over-dependence on the periodic reporting on programme progress by the grant sub-recipients. In the case of Zimbabwe, limited first-hand programme information has at times made it difficult for the body to make informed, evidence-based programme decisions and policies. Although such bodies are not expected to provide direct services to the public, the perspective of the Global Fund's beneficiaries is important. Rights-based HIV/AIDS programming requires the consultation and participation of those infected and/or affected by the virus in the construction of the programmes and activities. Whilst the Global Fund project proposal development processes are coordinated by the CCM, the exercise largely remains exclusive rather than inclusive with a greater involvement of technocrats whether from the public, private or civil society in drawing up these proposals. The CCM Secretariat's principal role is to provide administrative services to the CCM board through the provision of coordination, communication and networking, information sharing and secretarial support. This is often difficult as a result of limited resources and the absence of an operating budget. The revitalised CCM Sub-Committee on HIV/AIDS consists of technocrats delegated to address programme issues, inform and provide technical advice on Global Fund programme policy gaps to the CCM.

Mechanisms for grassroots participation in the CCM are not developed. These would allow the grassroots communities to participate in the identification of their HIV/AIDS programme needs, prioritisation, allocation of resources, implementation, monitoring and evaluation of the programme. A CCM oversight plan would equally allow the CCM to evaluate the impact of programmes for gender equality. Best judged by the undertaking of Global Fund expenditure studies, beneficiary assessments, and other qualitative and quantitative assessments using gender-sensitive indicators. In order to implement HIV/AIDS programmes that are effective and efficient, it is necessary to address the needs of the people in proposal development, and subsequently those in programme implementation, monitoring and evaluation.

The full participation and voices of CCM PLWHAs and female members remains weak, limiting any meaningful input into the Global Fund proposal development, resource distribution and CCM oversight activities. The meaningful participation of these groups could ensure that budgeted funds find their way to the point of service delivery, and that services operate in ways that respect human rights – especially of the poor and marginalised communities and groups – whilst ensuring that services are operated in ways that improves their lives. Low participation levels are evidenced by women's inability to voice their concerns, advocate for their rights, influence the CCM policy and decision-making processes, and challenge their male counterparts in a CCM environment dominated by male professionals. Inadequate programme and disease information, intertwined with gendered societal expectations also form major hurdles to full participation, with the recognition of traditional institutions still problematic in exercising women's rights (SARDC-WIDSAA 2000). In the case of PLWHAs, many policy-makers also remain convinced that they should receive services and have no business in the resource decision-making arena, coupled with the inferiority complex instilled in many PLWHAs, this makes the situation even more complex (UNNGLS 2001)

The CCM NGO representatives are expected to play an important role in ensuring participatory democracy by acting as a 'watchdog' with regards to the programme processes, including the undertaking of general assessments of the quantity, quality and appropriateness of the public service delivery. There is limited evidence of the added value of local NGO participation in the CCM. NGOs play a vital role in strengthening democracy and good governance through representation of different voices, perspectives and values. Their behaviour was in contrast to the CCM members from the international non-governmental organisations, who represented some of the external and direct funders of the Global Fund funding mechanism from the European Union and the United States. This group was more vocal and exhibited higher levels of the independence and autonomy that are cited as preconditions for participation. The inclusion of sub-recipients within the CCM at times results in a CCM quorum with special and narrow interests that are capable of driving the agenda in protection of their interests and with a potential for conflicts of interest.

There are CCM private sector representatives as full members of the CCM, though the benefit of PPP in Zimbabwe has yet to be realised as a result of the harsh economic environment. In a vibrant economy, the private sector can play an important role through the augmentation of public sector and donor resources. The private sector level of participation in CCM meetings appeared largely hindered by limited access and availability to Global Fund programme information, CCM governance tools, instruments, and general misconceptions and lack of clarity surrounding the CCM 'governance versus management roles.' Politics of professional dominance often resulted in minimal relevant discourse on programme governance issues. Discussions were usually overly concentrated on programme issues, distracting members from their governance role. The CCM governance role should include the determination of in-country policy and strategies, active monitoring of the grant performance, managing the governance process, and providing the principal recipients with much needed insight, wisdom and judgment. There is a need for the development of mechanisms and/or strategies for increased CCM interaction and consultation with its external local stakeholders importantly decentralised grant recipients and beneficiaries.

Zimbabwe is unique in that, up to December 2007, it had two principal recipients of Global Fund grants: the UNDP and the NAC. Whilst both organisations are equally suited as principal recipients, the NAC 'understudied' UNDP. UNDP has notable strengths that include a strong operational backbone, orientation and processes that enable results-based programming, financial planning and management capacities and resources to employ international management standards. It remains a centralised and bureaucratic structure that allows for minimal participation of external stakeholders including those affected and infected by the virus. The NAC, however, continues to refine its development interventions through rigorous analysis, shared knowledge and consultation with programmatic partners. The Global Fund budget is limited to social mobilisation and advocacy activities. In contrast the NAC, with its decentralised structures and management of the Global Fund programme's coordination component, is able to engage regularly with various programme implementers through planned quarterly coordination and review meetings.

NAC and UNDP jointly undertake decentralised quarterly support, monitoring, evaluation, data validation, sub-recipient and sub-sub-recipient, verification and internal audit field activities. In the absence of a strong civil society that exerts pressure from outside, or below, on policy-making elites, full participation of all stakeholders remains limited (Healey and Robinson, 1993). Mechanisms are not fully developed to receive programme complaints or provide timely programme information and feedback to the grant implementers. The principal recipients meet regularly with the CCM and sub-recipients, and provide updated programme progress reports, though the principal recipients have limited contact with sub-sub-recipients.[16] The principal recipient's grant roles and responsibilities are clearly defined in various Global Fund/ UNDP and or UNDP/NAC programme documentation and letters of agreement. These also include programme management; grant (resource) management (including periodic disbursement of funds, materials and support for programme human resources) and accounting, programme supervision, monitoring, evaluation, and undertaking of internal audits, documentation and reporting. The principal recipients, sub-recipients and sub-sub-recipients are not always present at, or invited to, the CCM proposal development and finalisation processes, and are often requested to implement programmes and plans where they have had minimal involvement or participation in the programme, project design or conceptualisation stages. This results in conflicting ownership issues, and highlights the need for regular staff social mobilisation and advocacy, as result of continuing high staff attrition in the key decentralised implementation levels.

The sub-recipients and sub-sub-recipients mainly consist of civil society organisations including faith-based organisations.[17] The NAC is also a principal recipient and a grant sub-recipient. Its role is to coordinate the Global Fund inputs and jointly monitor and evaluate the Global Fund programme. This important group contributes to the attainment of Global Fund indicators, targets, and the direct and indirect provision of HIV/AIDS services as according to the implementation plan. Though NGOs are chosen as grant recipients because of their decentralised structures and proximity to the grassroots there is minimal evidence that the grassroots potential is being harnessed through active participatory engagement and dialogue mechanisms. In a conducive operating environment, this serves to broaden discussions on organisational policies, strategies and operational issues. In all examples cited above institutional transparency – involving the provision of accessible and timely information to stakeholders and the opening up of organisational procedures, structures and processes for their assessment – remain governance challenges. It was reported by Global Fund stakeholders that rigid and inflexible Global Fund contractual obligations, with limited budgetary allocations for communication and information sharing and exchange activities, makes stakeholder communication difficult. Grant implementers were constrained by soaring inflation and the unplanned need for increased local resources for the production of information, education and communication training materials as people's education was essential for their full and knowing participation. Where possible, periodic NATF inputs to the decentralised NAC structures served to augment GFATM budget allocations in this regard.

Global Fund institutional accountability

The LFA is solely accountable to the Global Fund in Geneva; although this is largely perceived as being at the expense of in-country stakeholders and grant beneficiaries. Whilst organisations cannot be equally accountable to all internal and external stakeholders, particular key stakeholders need to be prioritised when taking into account factors such as influence, responsibility and representation.[18] With minimal public information on the modus operandi of this body, and the terms of reference unknown to the Global Fund stakeholders, the need for greater accountability remains an essential element in improving institutional system performance. However, there are different forms of accountability, which depend on different types (administrative, financial, and political) and directions (horizontal, downwards, upwards) of accountability relations. LFA accountability relations are largely upwards.

The LFA as a key decision- and policy-maker with respect to in-country Global Fund grant awarding, operations, and management should be held accountable by the grant beneficiaries, institutional stakeholders and the public at large. Particular reference is made, for example, to the controversies that surrounded the Global Fund denial of several Zimbabwean grants applications for HIV/AIDS, tuberculosis, and malaria over the years and unexplained grant suspension in Round One. Blagescu *et al.* argue that an accountable organisation should be transparent, involve all in key decision-making processes related to practice and policies, evaluate performance, policies and practice in consultation, learns and reports on outputs (Blagescu *et al.* 2005). Whereas the CCM is directly accountable to the Government of Zimbabwe, it is also indirectly accountable to the bilateral and multilateral funding of the Global Fund. It is not clear to whom the local sector CCM members are accountable, as it is difficult to determine whether sectoral representatives of the CCM do in fact report within their sectors, what form this feedback takes, or which communication channels and/or tools are used. The lack of feedback from CCM membership constituencies influences the level of knowledge and CCM member debate and their participation in this governance body. Effective accountability requires information; and scrutiny is not possible unless those who might scrutinise public actions are well informed about them (UNDP 2006). Though CCM members are requested to share information between them, several representatives cited communication challenges. CCM debates and discussions are circulated by the CCM Secretariat but not for public consumption, as evident in the absence of public communications in the local media. The general public requires information about the performance of their CCM representatives and the CCM body if they are to hold them and the institution accountable. Information will influence the quality of its governance in the absence of structural mechanisms that could enable the general public to interact with the CCM and influence its agenda. The quality of CCM outputs and service were further compromised due to a lack of clear definition between the CCM governance roles and the principal recipient's management roles, adequate and updated information on the grant progress and familiarity of their own governance instruments, again seen to compromise the quality of debate and discussion.

UNDP, as the principal recipient, is directly accountable to the Global Fund as specified in the contractual agreement between the two organisations, and indirectly accountable for the financial and programme management to the CCM and the LFA. The CCM exhibited transparency through ensuring that the principal recipients provide Global Fund programme information and updates in its regular meetings. These reports consisted of Global Fund programme management progress, challenges and constraints with particular reference to the Global Fund targets/indicators. The principal recipient presents verified and validated quarterly and annual grant financial, audit and programme progress reports with quarterly disbursement requests to the Global Fund in Geneva via the LFA. Following internal and external audits commissioned and supervised by the principal recipient, the principal recipient is obliged to report and provide feedback to all recipients.[19] Effective accountability is enhanced through the principal recipient's access to relevant, appropriate and timely dissemination of Global Fund and UNDP programme-related information, and these are communicated in a bid to enhance sub-recipient compliance, accountability and transparency related to resource management practices. For public consumption the principal recipient provides programme inputs to the UNDP Zimbabwe HIV/AIDS website, although the responses are not regularly evaluated. This mode of communication is limited to those with internet access. UNDP seeks to ensure that the implementing partners are trained and sensitised on the use of the available Global Fund programme governance tools and instruments such as programme and financial policies, guidelines, protocols and manuals.

Whilst the NAC is directly accountable to the Ministry of Health and Child Welfare, the NAC Board, and indirectly accountable to every worker and business who pays the AIDS levy and corporate tax. Further indirect accountability of the NAC is to all beneficiaries of the NATF. The organisation accountability relations are generally upwards to the NAC Board and Ministry of Health and Child Welfare in relation to administrative, financial, and political accountability.

Though with weak accountability, monitoring and evaluation practices it remains difficult to categorically state that resources indeed meet the needs of the intended HIV/AIDS grant (Global Fund and/or NATF) beneficiaries. A 2007 Institute for Security and Transparency International Zimbabwe report on South Africa's HIV/AIDS response cited that corruption and poor management hampers the fight against HIV/AIDS. The massive government and donor inflow of funds reportedly has little effect in halting the epidemic. In the examination of accountability within the national and provincial levels, the report cited a host of problems in the management of resources allocated to fighting the disease. These included poor budgetary management and execution or poor 'budget tracking mechanisms', especially with regards to donor funding. Lack of accountability and transparency is evident in regards to financial management, massive under-spending by lower levels and decentralised structures, and growing concerns over the institutional processes for the spending of HIV /AIDS funding. In the conclusion of the report it was stated that the 'more loose and unregulated the system, the greater the chance of corruption.' This report should be a cause for concern in Zimbabwe in light of the weakening of HIV /AIDS national institutions and decentralised structures with the continuing economic decline. The NAC decentralised structures at the district level – which are key pillars for the Global Fund and NATF resource planning, allocation and service delivery – have been hard hit by an exodus of qualified staff.

Most sub-recipients are concentrated in the capital city of Harare, with branches in other larger towns whilst providing Global Fund outreach services in twelve far flung rural and remote districts. This situation has the potential of minimising the sub-recipient financial and programmatic oversight role aimed at improving the sub-sub-recipient's quality of governance.

Limited decentralisation, devolution of roles, responsibility, and decision-making, affect grant implementation, support, monitoring and evaluation. Due to resource constraints, sub-recipients have limited contact with their sub-sub-recipients, thereby also limiting the amount and quality of accessible and timely information passing through these decentralised implementing structures, to partners and intended beneficiaries.

Sub-sub-recipients are formally contracted by sub-recipients to provide decentralised services to the grassroots communities and also act as lower level decision and policy makers. There is limited accountability to their HIV/AIDS service recipients as a result of cited logistical and communication difficulties. The current sub-sub-recipient contract arrangement precludes accountability to the principal recipient except via the sub-recipient, which occurs in the form of quarterly financial and programme progress reports. Internal and external sub-recipient audits are conducted once a year in which examination of revenues and expenditures are made, so as to ensure that sub-recipients maintain accounting records, documents and other evidence relating to the programme grant agreement. In general limited accountability by sub-recipients and sub-sub-recipients to their constituencies may have been as a result of marginalisation of the grassroots population in their own institutional operations. Sub-sub-recipients face accountability challenges as a result of their inability to respond to lower level and community views, concerns and needs. This becomes apparent in their limited local participation, knowledge of Global Fund operational information, and no participation in the national decision making processes and structures. There is need to build stronger and more responsive accountability frameworks, budgeting systems, to facilitate much needed timely disbursements and enhancement of absorptive capacities. Low compliance rates are attributed to high staff attrition and poor institutional memories within the decentralised structures, necessitating the need for regular institutional and individual capacity building and strengthening initiatives following periodic capacity assessments. Lack of a sense of ownership of Global Fund interventions affects transparency, accountability and participation as good governance norms.

Responsiveness as another key feature of good governance requires all the NAC and Global Fund institutions to provide accessible, available, and affordable access to HIV/AIDS prevention (including new information), treatment, care and mitigation services particularly targeting PLWHAs and other marginalised groups (including women). This can only occur if obliging Global Fund actors respond with a variety of tools and approaches, and requires the participatory involvement of all people and influential others in the decentralised HIV/AIDS service delivery, policy formulation and implementation structures. This will ensure sustainability of HIV and AIDS multi-sectoral long-term responses cited in the Zimbabwe National Strategic HIV and AIDS Plan of 2006.

Accountable structures need to increasingly take proactive rather than reactive steps to address needs of stakeholders, become transparent in activities and decision making processes, and engage in on-going dialogue, to enable them to make informed decisions, related to policies and practice. Evaluations of Global Fund grant performance, policies and practice should be undertaken in consultation with key stakeholders and enable organisations and related structures to learn from and report on outputs of these evaluations on a regular basis. Organisations require channels through which stakeholders can voice their grievances and receive appropriate responses. Thus placing increased emphasis on two-way communication and reporting by Global Fund internal and external stakeholders on resource management, and undertaking of financial monitoring activities. The conducting of relevant and appropriate reporting on the HIV/AIDS programme outcomes, following internal and external audits, strengthens Global Fund institutional accountability and oversight roles, and provides assurance that resources are being properly used. Where there is free flow of information about public affairs, this enables citizens to engage in debate and discussion about leading issues of the day, resulting in competent citizens who will not tolerate abuse of resources. The use of different media should be seen as key to securing and enhancing accountability within Global Fund structures and amongst beneficiaries.

Conclusion

This chapter discussed the role of the local funding mechanism of the NATF and the complementary Global Fund funding structures in conjunction with institutional governance norms and practices namely participation, accountability, transparency and responsiveness as essential for the efficient and effective delivery of HIV/AIDS resources and services. Concern was expressed at the varying degrees institutional accountability and transparency with regards to the administration of HIV/AIDS funds, distribution of ARVs and the worsening plight of the people living with HIV/AIDS under the declining economic conditions where corruption is fast becoming a norm.

Whilst Zimbabwe is a country in difficult circumstances, good governance practices for sustained inflow of resources for the HIV/AIDS response rests on the power, ability and means to communicate and obtain feedback from stakeholders and influential others. Recognition of donor grant conditionalties and a partnership approach is needed so as to enhance mutual trust between funders, recipients and beneficiaries. Notably communication for development will remain an integral part, though often underplayed and poorly resourced, to sustain and address good governance norms and characteristics (Panos 2007). The United Nations Human Development Report in 2001 states that good governance is dependent on effective information systems and addressing communication challenges. Strong governance institutions and broad based participation in the development process can improve the effectiveness of the AIDS response (UNDP 2007). Accountability should not only be to funders, stakeholders, legal authorities, the state, and selective groupings but importantly to the intended programme beneficiaries through organisational and institutional frameworks which each person can contribute towards development of solutions to their problems. Whilst fiscal decentralisation as in the case of the NAFT and the Global Fund structures seeks to enhance accountability, and ownership, there is need for support for institutional and individual capacity building and effective HIV/AIDS management and implementation, oversight activities at the lower levels. Participation can only be achieved if all local and international actors in the HIV/AIDS multisectional response are willing and, importantly, able to contribute to the various structures and processes. Enabling participation requires education and mobilisation of service providers and users through different communication, monitoring and feedback processes (Panos 2007).

For a sustained Zimbabwean HIV/AIDS multisectoral response in light of the harsh operating socioeconomic environment and declining internal and external funding base, there is need for national recognition, in order to address the emerging governance challenges. The strengthening of the existing institutional good governance practices requires the internalisation of these practices as processes rather than events or conditions precedent for continued resource inflows, together with greater involvement of all infected and affected people in the making of decisions that affect their livelihoods in an increasingly transparent and accountable manner. Global Fund and other external donor support are needed for the strengthening of institutional governance monitoring and evaluation processes and where necessary development of minimum institutional governance standards and tools based on the outcome of institutional appraisals.

Periodic assessments should be undertaken of the quality of the governance information systems, and these should form the basis for building capacities in governance monitoring, and allow for governments, CCMs in particular and other Global Fund structures to better prioritize, monitor and develop governance indicators. Accessible, available, user friendly and timely information pertaining to the HIV/AIDS multisectoral institutional responses, together with increased openness and public and private media reporting around organisational procedures, structures and processes for assessment, heightens the level of transparency and reduces the potential for corrupt practices in an increasingly resource constrained environment. Information will enable the general public to judge whether the local policies are being properly implemented and hold the NAC, NAFT and Global Fund accountable on promises made. The development and utilisation of institutional governance tools and instruments further enhances good governance practices and increase levels of public debate. Red tape should be set aside around public goods and service delivery and allow for the examination of public accounts including the NATF and Global Fund grants outside of the formal structures such as the CCM. It is important that the national, NATF and Global Fund structures and development funds are accountable to their beneficiaries and as these are public funds and resources, must be able to stand up to scrutiny.

Notes

1 The cited good governance principles include accountability, transparency, leadership and management, participation, effective partnership building, representation, decentralisation of power and institutional responsiveness to mandate.

2 Three major events signaled as far back as 2005 that financial support for international remedial efforts against HIV/AIDS faced an uncertain future. A UNAIDS report cited a funding gap 2005–7; the Global Fund identified funding gap of US $700 million in 2005 and stated that it was unlikely that the WHO sationwill succeed in a stated goal to provide 3 million people with ARV treatment by 2005 in resource-poor countries. In 2005, a G8 communiqué from rich nations resolved to hold recipient countries accountable for verifiable progress in governance and anti-corruption measures and stated that they were likely not to redeem their pledges of additional financial assistance to recipient countries deemed lacking in governance.

3 Participation: The process through which an organisation enables stakeholders to play an active role in the decision-making processes and activities, which affect them. The Global Accountability Project (GAP) alludes to participation as an important dimension of accountability. Participation should not be confined to the centrally resource rich level but, should filter down at the most immediate level of governance the grassroots level, where the general populaces encounter the effects of economic and social policies, and the various laws and health and development programmes. Arnstien (1969) also states that participation should include supporting, acting together, deciding together, consultation and provision of information.

4 Transparency involves providing accessible, appropriate and timely information to stakeholders and the opening up of organisational procedures, structures and processes for public assessment. It focuses on making systems and processes accountable to all users, stakeholders and is not confined to a privileged few. It is about the level of openness of the institution, provision of information for all to make informed decisions about its operations and provide a benchmark from where the organisation can be judged as conforming to set standards, levels, performance and targets.

5 Organisational responsiveness addresses the ability of an institution to respond to stakeholders concerns and needs and its ability to take heed and adjust policies, programmes and intended interventions accordingly. As such, being accountable is about being open and engaging in ongoing dialogue. This improves the level of programme ownership and sustainability.

6 Accountability relates to the process through which an organissation makes a commitment to respond to and balance the needs of stakeholders in its decision-making processes and activities, and delivers against its commitment. Monitoring for accountability is crucial using indicators (structural, process and outcome) as a monitoring tool.

7 A Private paper, *The Zimbabwe Financial Gazette* November 29–December 5, 2007.

8 National AIDS Council of Zimbabwe Act 15.14 and Section 30 of the Audit and Exchequer Act Chapter 22:03.

9 Mkandwire, T. and Soludo, C. (1999). *Our Continent, Our Future*, Dakar: Codesria and IDRC

10 Zimbabwe adopted a multi-sectoral response to HIV and AIDS and upholds the 'Three Ones' initiative, which stipulates that there must be:

- one coordinating authority (the NAC);
- one strategic framework (the Zimbabwe HIV and Aids Strategic Plan, 2006–10); and
- one national monitoring and evaluation system (which is administered by NAC).

11 A presentation by D. Muchemwa LFA Representative at the Regional Meeting for Southern African 'Sharing Innovative Solutions for Enhanced Program Delivery", Windhoek. Namibia, 8–10 May 2007.

12 Reference is made to paragraph 34 and 35. Fifth Board Meeting Geneva, 5–6 June 2003 and the Revised Guidelines on the Purpose, Structure and Composition of the Country Coordinating Mechanisms and Requirements for Grant Eligibility – Incorporating CCM related decisions 10th Board Meeting, Geneva April 2005.

13 The CCM has fiduciary arrangements and local governance instruments including a Terms of Reference (January 2005), Ethics and Conflict of Interest Policy (August 2005), Rules of Procedure (January 2005) and Guide for Consistency Member Selection to the Zimbabwe CCM document.

14 Ownership also involves accountability, with different types of accountability to different stakeholders.

15 Related to the processes through which the organisation, with involvement of stakeholders, monitors and reviews its progress and results against goals and objectives, feeds learning back to the organisation on an ongoing basis; and reports on the results of the process.

16 This diverse group had different mandates, structures, internal processes, responsibilities (mission, goals, objectives and philosophies), and governance tools and instruments. For attainment of the GFATM objectives there was need for institutional education and harmonisation with the PR UNDPs' governance tools and instruments. These included the UNDP Manual for projects financed by the Global Fund to fight AIDS, Tuberculosis, and Malaria, UNDP Financial Regulations and rules, UNDP Procurement Manual, Imprest Account guidelines, UNDP Programming Manual, Administrative Circular Number: 2006/2009 Accountability, Transparency and Results management and Guidelines for processing VAT Refund claims. Programme guidance was contained in the exchange of letters between Global Fund and UNDP Headquarters of 16–17 December 2003 and Government of Zimbabwe and UNDP.

17 Failure to understand influence as not only power can affect the already skewed accountability systems towards those with power at the expense of those without power, in this case the other GFATM governance structures in country and intended grant beneficiaries at the grassroots level.

Bibliography

A Private paper, *The Zimbabwe Financial Gazette* November 29–December 5 2007.

Abuja Declaration on HIV/AIDS, Tuberculosis and other related Infectious Diseases (2000). Abuja, Nigeria.

Agere, S. (1998). *Zimbabwe Post–Independence Public Administration: Management Policy Issues and Constraints*, Dakar: CODESRIA.

Akukwe, C. (2005). *H.I.V./AIDS: Looming Funding Crisis*, Worldpress.org, Online. Available http://www.worldpress.org/Africa/2123.cfm – 48k (Accessed 1 June 2006).

Arnstein, S. (1969). A Ladder of Citizen Participation, *JAIP*, Vol. 35, No. 4.

Blagescu, M., de las Casas, L. and Lloyd, R. (2005). *Pathways to Accountability – A short Guide to GAP Framework*, One World Trust, United Kingdom.

Byanyima, W. (2000). Parliamentary Governance and Gender Budgeting: the Ugandan Experience in United Nations Development Fund for Women (UNIFEM), *Gender Budget Initiatives. Strategies, Concepts and Experiences*, New York: UNIFEM.

Central Statistical Office (CSO) (2006). *Zimbabwe Demographic Health Survey 2005–2006*, Government of Zimbabwe: Harare.

Cheema, W. (2005). *Building Democratic Institutions: Governance Reform in Developing Countries*, Sterling, VAT: Kumarian Press.

Global Fund to Fight AIDS, Tuberculosis and Malaria (2007). *Country Coordinating Mechanisms*, Geneva: GFATM.

Hatendi, F. and Makondo, E. (2003). *An Examination of the Institutional Arrangements Established to Address the Challenges of HIV/AIDS in Zimbabwe*, unpublished, Harare: Idasa.

Healey, J. and Robinson, M. (1993). *Democracy, Governance and Economic Policy*, London: ODI.

Joint United Nations Programme on HIV/AIDS (UNAIDS). (2005). *Evidence for HIV decline in Zimbabwe: A comprehensive review of the epidemiological data*, UNAIDS/05.26E.

MDGD/UNDP (2000). Decentralised Governance: A Global Matrix of Experiences, New York: UNDP.

Ministry of Health and Child Welfare (2007). Zimbabwe National HIV/AIDS Estimates, Harare.

Ministry of Finance (MoF) (1999). Audit and Exchequer Act, Chapter 22:03, Section 30. Government Printers, Zimbabwe.

Mkandwire, T. and Soludo, C. (1999). *Our Continent, Our Future*, Dakar: CODESRIA and IDRC.

Moyo, S., Makumbe, J. and Raftopoulos, B. (2000). NGOs; the State & Politics in Zimbabwe, Harare: SAPES Books.

National AIDS Council (2007). *Zimbabwe National HIV/AIDS Strategic Plan*, Government Printers, Harare.

National AIDS Council of Zimbabwe Act (NAC) (2001). Chapter: 14 No 16/99, Government Printers, Harare.

Nwanma, V. (2001). Africa puts fight against AIDS at fore front, *Africa Recovery*, Vol.15 (1–2): 6–8.

Panos (2007). *The Case for Communication in Sustainable Development, Promoting dialogue, debate and change*, London.

Poku, N. and McGrew, A. (2007). *Social Citizenship and Governance*, UBC Press.

SADC (2000). *Regional Human Development Report*, UNDP/SADC/SAPES TRUST, Harare.

SARDC-WIDSAA (2000). *Inequalities Women in Southern Africa*, SARDC, Harare.

Strode, A. and Grant, K. (2004). *Understanding the institutional dynamics of South Africa's response to the HIV/AIDS pandemic*, Institute for Democracy in South Africa (IDASA)

The Global Fund to Fight AIDS, Tuberculosis and Malaria. (2004). *Country Coordinating Mechanisms – Building Good Governance*, Discussion paper, Geneva.

The Standard Supplement World AIDS Day 25 November 2000.

The University of Warwick and UNDP (2007). Working *Paper 2, National Governance and HIV/AIDS Responses*, Warwick: CSGR.

Transparency International – Zimbabwe (2007). *Calling for Transparency and Accountability in HIV/AIDS*, Harare.

UN (2001). Declaration of Commitment on HIV/AIDS, United Nations General Assembly Special Session on HIV/AIDS, New York.

UNAIDS (2007). *Financial Resources required to achieve universal access to HIV prevention, treatment, care and support,* GRNE Advisory Board Meeting, Geneva.

UNAIDS/UNDP Governance of HIV/AIDS Responses: Issues and Outlook, New York, UNDP.

UNDP (1997). *Governance for Sustainable Human Development*-A UNDP Policy document, New York, UNDP.

—— (2000). Zimbabwe *Human Development Report*, Harare, UNDP.

—— (2002). Special Issue: Technical Cooperation, *Development Policy Journal*, 2:73–94, NewYork: UNDP.

UNDP Regional Bureau for Africa. (2006) *Strategy and Management Review*, New York, UNDP.

UNNGLS (2001). *Voices from Africa to NGO Responses to HIV/AIDS*, Geneva.

UN General Assembly (UNGASS) (2006). *Report on HIV and AIDS Zimbabwe Country Report* UN: Geneva.

WHO (2005). *Zimbabwe,* Geneva, Switzerland.

8 The causes, contours and consequences of the multisectoral response to HIV/AIDS

Sophie Harman

If only they had listened.[1]

Anon, non-governmental organisation, Kenya

We remind them ruthlessly that, no, you are a politician, you are not the mechanics ... you know very well you are a public representative, your objective is this.[2]

Nadeem Mohammed, AIDS Campaign Team Africa, World Bank

A central mechanism for making governance of the HIV/AIDS response more participatory and accountable to people living with and affected by the epidemic has been the introduction of a multisectoral approach. The socio-economic determinants of HIV/AIDS within countries with high prevalence rates require a varied and disaggregated response to the epidemic that encompasses all aspects of society – from teachers, religious leaders and local government, to the international organisations and donors that fund their projects. The need to adopt this approach, and to encourage other aspects of society to participate in tackling the spread of HIV/AIDS underpins the concept of multisectorality: the idea that to fight HIV/AIDS, you need to involve all of society.

This chapter looks at the origin of multisectorality, and how it has been harnessed and promoted by the World Bank as a means of participatory governance in the response to the HIV/AIDS epidemic. It will unravel some of the contradictions and problems with this approach in practice, what this means for accountable and participatory governance of HIV/AIDS, and how we can understand the role of international organisations and processes of global governance through the World Bank. The chapter does so by looking at the impact of the Bank's Multi-Country AIDS Programme (MAP) with specific reference to Kenya, Tanzania and Uganda.[3] It pursues this aim by first explaining what the World Bank means by multisectorality, and why and how the Bank has come to occupy a central role within HIV/AIDS governance. Second, the chapter briefly builds on Chapter 4 of this book, by explaining the contours of multisectorality within the MAP. Third, the chapter discusses some of the successes and limitations of the Bank's approach to multisectorality in promoting participation and accountability. In so doing, it draws together the consequences of multisectorality on the HIV/AIDS response in conclusion.

Causes: Multisectorality and the World Bank

Prior to the emergence of the multisectoral approach, the response to HIV/AIDS was firmly located within the discipline of public health, led by the World Health Organisation (WHO)'s Global Programme on HIV/AIDS (GPA). The GPA, under the leadership of Jonathan Mann, recognised the non-health implications of the epidemic and the role of non-governmental organisations (NGOs) within this, but it was not until the United Nations Development Programme (UNDP) articulated the need to address the long-term causes of HIV/AIDS towards the late 1980s that the concept of multisectorality entered the global discourse. UNDP's interpretation of multisectorality during this period referred to the need to recognise the socioeconomic dynamics of the epidemic, the problems it poses for developing countries, and to link the epidemic more widely to development policy within international organisations and member states. Operationally, this recognition has led to UNDP engaging with both health and non-health specific actors as a means of addressing issues such as gender and stigma, and incorporating the non-health aspects of HIV/AIDS within government strategies to address the epidemic (UNDP 2008).

Despite UNDP initially articulating the need for multisectorality during the late 1980s, it was not until 15 years later, when the World Bank encompassed the concept within its flagship HIV/AIDS project for Sub-Saharan Africa – the MAP – that the term became widely applied. The MAP was a US$1 billion project that would provide funding to any country in Sub-Saharan Africa that has a strategic plan to fight HIV/AIDS, would ensure to distribute 40–60 per cent of the funds it received to non-state actors, and has a national coordinating body. It was launched in 2000, and currently operates in 30 countries. The central working practices of the Bank have come to underpin the global response to HIV/AIDS (Harman, 2007). What is crucial about the MAP is how it interprets multisectorality – and thus participation and accountability – in line with the Bank's approach to development.

For the Bank, multisectorality very much referred to the need to encompass all aspects of society within the response to HIV/AIDS, but principally those working in the community that educate people on methods of prevention, and care for the sick and their families. The MAP would empower these people by providing them with financial support, and encourage the governments of states to respond to the challenge of HIV/AIDS accordingly by establishing national AIDS councils that would provide a crucial coordination and leadership role (World Bank 2000a–f; 2001; 2003a–e; 2007e). The national AIDS councils would then establish local district and community AIDS councils to work directly with the community and disburse MAP funds to them. The national AIDS council structures thus became the working mechanisms of the MAP and the Bank; as Hayes suggests in Chapter 4 of this book, the National AIDS Control Council (NACC) in Kenya, became the Bank's 'eyes and ears' in that country.

What is specific about the Bank's interpretation of multisectorality is its clear relationship to the ideological shifts within the Bank during the 1990s. Up until the introduction of the MAP, the Bank had not developed any global HIV/AIDS programmes. HIV/AIDS was included within the wider remit of sexual health programmes, and country-specific projects in Brazil, India and Zimbabwe. Further to these specific projects, the Bank had started to conduct research into the epidemic with the release of its 1997 report *Confronting AIDS: public priorities in a global epidemic*, which considered how the Bank should move forward within the sphere of HIV/AIDS. The Bank also entered into joint initiatives with UN agencies in its role as a co-sponsor of UNAIDS. The most common explanation as to the origins of the MAP and the Bank's subsequent take on multisectorality was the role of two key staff members – Debrework Zewdie and Hans Binswanger. Binswanger, an AIDS activist within the Bank, was committed to community-driven development. Zewdie was an Ethiopian doctor who worked on public health and has witnessed the affect of HIV/AIDS upon Sub-Saharan Africa. Combined, the two brought the problem of HIV/AIDS to the Bank's Board of Directors, and convinced them that the Bank had to act on the problem for the following reasons: (i) HIV/AIDS is a development problem and the Bank is a development agency; (ii) the Bank prioritises community-driven development and the HIV/AIDS response is centred on community-driven development; and (iii) the Bank had so far done very little on HIV/AIDS (*Int.* Zewdie 2006). Three months after approaching the Board of Directors, Zewdie, Binswanger and three other members of staff drafted the MAP. The Board agreed for the MAP to be an adaptable programme loan, whereby the Bank would commit US$ 1billion and the vice-president for the region would then approve individual programmes for individual countries. This was intended to speed up the process of getting the money to the ground.

The agency of Binswanger and Zewdie in getting the Bank to concentrate on HIV/AIDS, specifically from a multisectoral approach, should not be underestimated. However, it ignores the wider institutional dynamics of the time, which have ultimately shaped how the Bank has defined multisectorality, applied it to the global response to HIV/AIDS, and impacted upon governance, participation and accountability. The MAP's form of multisectorality encapsulates the central features of World Bank President James Wolfensohn's (1995–2005) reform package, and the emphasis placed on partnership, state ownership, sharing of knowledge and civil society inclusion. Upon his appointment on 16th March 1995, Wolfensohn emphasised a change in Bank philosophy that would focus upon development, aid and the relationship between the Bank and borrower countries (Stiglitz 2003: 122). The Bank sought to improve effectiveness through better managed and implemented projects, to create a more holistic partnership with borrowing countries and wider inclusion of civil society organisations (CSOs) as a means of promoting institutional and project transparency, participation and accountability. Each of these ideological principles were to be operationalised through the Comprehensive Development Framework (CDF) country-specific Poverty Reduction Strategy Papers (PRSPs) and the Heavily Indebted Poor Country Initiative (HIPC).

At the heart of each of these programmes was 'the interdependence of all elements of development', which recognises country ownership and the long-term aspect of development (World Bank 2007a). The PRSPs would be designed in partnership with borrowing governments, and would reflect a particular country's macroeconomic and social policies, and reflect its financial needs (World Bank 2007b). Through processes such as the CDF and PRSPs, this era saw unprecedented levels of civil society integration within the Bank. Integration in this regard referred to consultation, dialogue, partnering and direct funding. Funding is either direct from the Bank's headquarters in Washington, through partnership with other donor agencies, community-driven development projects or specific projects such as the MAP (World Bank 2007c). These central components of the Wolfensohn reform agenda – country ownership, civil society partnership, accountability and transparency, and the need to take a holistic approach to development – underpin the MAP. It was the shift in approach under Wolfensohn that gave space for the MAP to be created and reflected the approach to multisectorality it takes. This can be seen in the following ways:

- Country ownership: All recipients of MAP funds should have a National AIDS Council (NAC) committed to multisectorality, that will lead and coordinate the national response to HIV/AIDS.
- Civil society participation: 40–60 per cent of funds must be channelled to CSOs, specifically community groups, in line with the Bank's commitment to community-driven development.
- The interdependence of development issues: A response to HIV/AIDS should be multisectoral in encompassing all aspects of and actors within society.
- Holistic approach to development: HIV/AIDS is a development issue, thus the Bank has a remit to act.

Thus for the Bank, multisectorality within HIV/AIDS governance has arisen in response to the institutional change of the late 1990s. Multisectorality has come to mean civil society participation that is located firmly within the community, and the involvement of all actors of society, under the leadership and governance of the national AIDS councils. In using the MAP to implement this form of multisectorality in 30 countries, the Bank has established both itself and its approach at the centre of HIV/AIDS governance. As the next section will show, this interpretation of multisectorality has become problematic for processes of participation and accountability within HIV/AIDS governance.

Contours Of multisectorality

Multisectorality through the MAP is expressed through two main contours: (i) partnership with governments through the national AIDS councils; and (ii) funding and dialogue with CSOs. This section will consider the practical elements of each of these two contours in turn.

Government partnership

The main contour of multisectorality is enhanced state and community participation through the centralised and localised structures of the NACs. The NACs are governmental bodies predominantly located within the president or prime minister's office, with the primary responsibility of coordinating the national response to HIV/AIDS and managing each country's respective MAP project. The NACs promote multisectorality through their management of the MAP by identifying those CSOs that should receive funds, strengthening their counterparts at the local level to work with community groups – i.e. the district and community AIDS councils – and working with international NGOs and international donors such as the Bank in the design of the national strategic plan. In so doing, the NACs are presented by the Bank as the owners of the MAP.[4] As local representatives of the NACs, the District AIDS Councils (DACs) promote multisectorality at the local level by funding community groups, coordinating the activities of multiple actors involved within the HIV/AIDS response at the local level, monitoring of MAP projects, and engaging feedback from community groups (National AIDS Control Council, 2005a-c; TACAIDS 2004; Uganda AIDS Commission 2004a–c; Uganda AIDS Commission 2005a–b).

The key role of these state bodies in promoting multisectorality is providing a bridge between the state and CSOs. The methods of CSO relations deployed by the NACs reflect the Bank's central approach to engagement: funding, dialogue and feedback, partnerships and networking (World Bank 2007c). Engagement with CSOs under the MAP principally refers to two types of CSO: (i) NGOs or faith-based organisations operating at the national level – this could refer to HIV/AIDS-specific organisations or groups such as the Girl Guides or organisations that specifically target private sector investment; and (ii) community groups operating within small specific geographical locations. CSO engagement through the structure of the governmental NAC/DAC structure is the basis for the Bank's brand of multisectorality. The role of the NACs and DACs presents the first contour of this; funding and dialogue between multiple actors provides the second contour of this.

Funding and dialogue

The main method of encouraging multisectoral participation within the HIV/AIDS response has been through the funding of CSOs with MAP funds. Funding to national NGOs is between US$ 14–25,000 and funding to community groups is US$ 1250 per annum (National AIDS Control Council 2005a; *Int.* Kiirya 2005). This funding is allocated, disbursed and monitored by the NAC/DAC government structure. Despite emphasising widespread participation within the multisectoral approach, the MAP does not fund international NGOs. The process of funding follows the pattern of:

- initial contact with local communities and community groups by targeting key members or leaders within a community;
- calls for proposals placed in mainstream and local press; and
- proposals submitted to either the DACs (if a community group) or the NACs (if an NGO operating nationally) for assessment. The assessment criteria are: the type of activity, duration, project and overhead costs, need, allocations of responsibility among staff.

The Bank does not become involved with the funding process or allocation of MAP resources unless applications are above US$25,000.

The multisectoral activities these groups engage in range from care and treatment, home-based care work, programmes for orphans and vulnerable children, psychosocial support for people infected with and affected by the disease, prevention, voluntary counselling and testing, mitigating the socio-economic impact of the epidemic, e.g. income-generating activities, and often a combination of all of the above. Research suggests that the majority of MAP funds disbursed to the community went to training programmes. For example, a community group would receive funds to train local members of the community in home-based care; these home-based carers would then train other members of the community, and so on. The problem with this, is that it often leads to a lack of delivery of services: groups are either training others or being trained, but are not actually using the skills that they have been trained in. Private sector activity under the MAP either refers to the development of specific HIV/AIDS programmes operating within private companies and businesses; targeting specific industries, e.g. taxi or bus driver associations, or engaging with business coalitions as a means of promoting HIV/AIDS programmes such as free anonymous testing at work, and educational networks (*Int.* Kataka 2005; *Int.* Gavyolea 2006). In response to the increased recognition of the feminisation of the epidemic, MAP programmes and multisectoral efforts target women-based NGOs and community groups, as well as ensuring the staff responsibilities of particular projects have an equal gender split.

Central to the MAP's approach to multisectorality is a commitment to open dialogue between all actors involved within the response, in which no-one is excluded (*Int.* Lagerstedt 16th November 2005). Dialogue in this regard takes the form of project feedback through report-writing, networking, quarterly meetings at community level, issue-based focus groups and national partnership meetings. Direct partnerships occur through joint planning meetings and operations. Unstructured forms of dialogue occur through community visits, and ad hoc meetings or activities. These forms of dialogue specifically pertain to the relationship between the government NAC/DAC system and the groups funded through the MAP.

The large number of actors involved within the multisectoral response promoted by the MAP makes it impossible to form a dialogue that includes everyone. This problem has been addressed by the introduction of networks. The formation of networks is encouraged by international donors such as the Bank and government agencies such as the NACs as a means of facilitating widespread participation, offering issue-specific expertise, and establishing direct links with the community (*Int.* Kalinga 2006). This recognition has seen a growth in networks and organisations seeking to group themselves under wider umbrella organisations with expanding mandates. Evidence of this can be seen in two regards: the rise of people living with HIV/AIDS (PLWHA) networks and networks of women's organisations.

Open dialogue permits a wider range of actors to engage in the MAP process, and hence greater multisectorality. This is specifically the case in regard to the inclusion of international NGOs who work within the government structures of the NACs and the health ministries. International NGOs participate within multisectoral responses through providing assistance in technical support, training institutions and implementation of key governmental strategies. As such, these NGOs are often evident within national strategic planning on the HIV/AIDS response, and are seen as an effective way to improve accountability and transparency within the governance process.

In sum, the contours of multisectorality within the MAP reflect similar processes of civil society engagement that are prioritised within the wider work of the Bank. The contours of engagement take the form of:

- funding, feedback and dialogue; and
- multisectoral activity organised around decentralised government structures – the NACs at the national level and the community AIDS councils or the DACs at the local level.

Consequences of multisectorality

Processes of multisectorality within the MAP have several consequences for the levels of participation and accountability it engenders. Similar to the contours of engagement, these consequences pertain to structures of funding and open dialogue, as well as division between different actors. This section explores each of these issues in turn, before considering how these consequences can be understood within the context of the Bank and global governance.

Funding and dialogue in practice

Participation within HIV/AIDS governance, through multisectoral processes such as the MAP, has been limited by delays in funding disbursal and lack of reciprocity in accountability measures. Widespread community opinion of organisations funded within the MAP in Kenya, Tanzania and Uganda suggested funding was too little, too late, and too short-term. Once the funding stopped, community multisectoral participation declined. There is a widespread opinion that, despite an awareness of funding being made available to small community groups, it is not in evidence on the ground.[5] Of those groups that received MAP funds, the need for monitoring and feedback mechanisms as a form of community and NGO accountability was seen as very demanding. Delays in funding, and the perception of high donor demand, challenge the inclusive, participatory nature of the multisectoral approach. In practice, multisectorality does not exist without the funding to implement it. This can be seen when looking at the consequences of multisectorality in regards to dialogue.

The methods of open dialogue created within the MAP only exist in terms of multisectoral funding. In practice, dialogue through report-writing and feedback is a form of holding community groups and NGOs to account, rather than a method of engaging their opinion and perspective on effective HIV/AIDS responses. This can be seen in the following ways. First, few community groups and NGOs sponsored under the MAP were involved in the initial design process of the project, or any broader national strategic plans. Consultation for both the MAP and strategic plans tended to occur in a consensual manner after the project was drawn up. Second, report-writing is a one-way process, with the NACs and DACs failing to reciprocate the structures of accountability to which community groups and NGOs must subscribe. As the NAC structures are governmental, this should not be problematic, because the government is an elective representative of the people; but this takes for the granted that the government was democratically elected, and that the NACs/DACs are not influenced by international donors and external factors. Established by the Bank, with the task of implementing the Bank's flagship project, and staffed by unelected civil servants, this cannot be taken for granted. Third, those organisations that are invited to participate in meetings, comment on strategic plans and engage directly with international donors, tend to form a group of similarly-minded organisations, well-versed in the language of HIV/AIDS governance. By this, they are able to use buzzwords such as 'multisectorality' 'good governance' and 'community participation' as well as comprehend the mass of acronyms used when talking about HIV/AIDS. Of the organisations interviewed that were participating in the MAP, some admitted to having prior relations with members of NACs, DACs or the Bank. These prior relations could be that they attended the same school (*Int.* Wambiya 2005), have staff members that previously worked or continued to work in these institutions, or acted as a consultant to the government prior to the MAP (*Int.* Otundo 2005; *Int.* Namatou 2005), or work for the Ministry of Health (*Int.* Talugende 2005). Prior relations were acknowledged as an important reason for their selection and subsequent participation.

The dominance of particular groups within funding and dialogue has led to division between actors participating within the multisectoral response. The organisations that have access to dialogue and decision-making tend to come from a select group of national and international NGOs. This access allows them to speak out about issues that affect communities, and thus re-enforce those structures that prevent communities speaking for themselves (*Int.* Okatcha 2005; *Int.* Maskika 2006). Compounding this is the relative advantage of international and national NGOs in having their headquarters in the capital cities, thus locating themselves closer to centres of decision-making (*Int.* Ngugi 2005). As multisectorality is generated through the funding of community activity, a high level of competition for resources exists between groups, which limits collaboration, cooperation and participation within the response. With one-sided accountability and limits to participation because of funding delays and restricted opportunities for feedback, frustration becomes a consequence of multisectorality, as opposed to widespread participation and open dialogue in HIV/AIDS governance. As such, we can see that multisectorality in practice, leads to the following consequences:

- funding delays that undermine participation;
- one-sided accountability measures;
- uneven dialogue structures;
- community frustration; and
- competition for resources and access to decision-making between actors.

Putting multisectorality in context

The causes and contours of multisectorality can very much be located within wider practices within the World Bank. Multisectorality through the implementation of the MAP in multiple countries in Sub-Saharan Africa arose out of: (i) the World Bank's approach to community-driven development and civil society organisation engagement practices; and (ii) the ability of key individuals within the Bank to harness this approach to comprehensive development and apply it to HIV/AIDS. These underpinnings of multisectorality have shaped the contours of the MAP in line with the Bank's main approach of civil society engagement and community-driven development – specific funding, structured forms of feedback and limited direct dialogue between the Bank and the groups that it funds. Relating the consequences of multisectorality to the Bank is not so clear. The consequences of multisectorality cannot necessarily be attributed directly to the Bank, however.

Delay in funding and problems of bureaucracy are an inevitable side effect of projects the size of the MAP; these issues were acknowledged in the project's initial design process, and measures were undertaken to reduce them as much as possible, i.e. making the MAP an adaptable programme loan. Difficulties in funding and dialogue are the responsibility of groups receiving funds as well as the Bank. However, the disaggregated structure of the MAP makes efforts to address these imbalances problematic. Key to these problems are discrepancies over ownership and direct dialogue that stem from the operational directives of the Bank's approach to community-driven development. The Bank does not directly engage with the groups that it funds because it is mandated to work with governments. In practice, this leads to one of the central contradictions of the MAP: on the one hand, the Bank absolves itself from responsibility or a leadership role in the project it funds, stressing the role of the NACs and governments as leaders of the national response; on the other hand, it makes MAP funds conditional on the government directing funds to CSOs, and articulating a specific form of national strategic plan that reflects the main tenets of the MAP.[6] The problem here lies in one-sided forms of accountability and participation: governments become accountable for the Bank's project through the NACs, but the Bank does not. Thus 'ownership', as expressed through the MAP and the Bank's wider projects means governments implementing the Bank's HIV/AIDS strategies, with little accountability on the part of the Bank, and little participation in articulating the HIV/AIDS agenda on the part of the NACs.

The discrepancy between NAC ownership and Bank conditionality is at the heart of the failure to fully engage with community groups and national NGOs under the MAP's multisectoral framework. Problems with engagement stem from an initial unwillingness of governments to engage with CSOs, and the lack of resources to do so. As engagement in this sense was initiated from the top-down, i.e. from the Bank, the NACs are in effect implementing the Bank's multisectoral approach with minimal real commitment on their own part. This is arguably changing with time and practice, but re-enforces the idea that in practice, multisectorality is more about participation through funding and programme implementation, and less about dialogue and decision-making. This form of multisectorality is thus both short-term and donor-driven. These two factors are recognised by the communities and national NGOs that receive MAP funds, and undermine the long-term vision of multisectorality held by the Bank and its partner international organisations. A consequence of multisectorality is thus not the long-term participation of multiple actors within the HIV/AIDS response, but a stop-gap measure that fails to address the long-wave nature of the epidemic. How multisectorality is expressed within the MAP does not fully engage in the type of multisectorality – full participation of all sectors of society – that the Bank and associated donors such as UNDP and UNAIDS set out to achieve.

The consequences of this become significantly problematic when considering the way in which UNAIDS, the Global Fund, UNDP, bilateral donors, and national governments have absorbed and prioritised this form of Bank-led multisectorality (Harman 2007). Community groups will continue to be involved in implementation-only engagement, and only select national NGOs will participate in consensual forms of dialogue. Pertinent issues such as gender and the feminisation of HIV/AIDS will not be fully addressed, as directives will come from the international organisations who are unaccountable to the people that their policies affect, and not from the communities in which change has to occur.

Conclusion

This chapter has begun to unravel a form of governance that is particular to HIV/AIDS: multisectorality. It has explained the concept of multisectorality as the process of stimulating widespread participation from all aspects of society in the response to HIV/AIDS. This concept stems from the notion that the socioeconomic causes and outcomes of the epidemic require multiple forms of intervention, from the education of young children to needle exchanges for intravenous drug users. At the centre of multisectorality is the role of community groups and national NGOs, as the most effective method of reaching every space within a country. The concept of multisectorality has been adopted by the World Bank and implemented through its MAP through the mass funding of small community groups, larger national NGOs, and the establishment of government agencies at the national, district and community level. Through the MAP, the Bank implemented a form of multisectorality that reflected the institution's approach to community-driven development at the time, which emphasised civil society participation, government ownership, and accountable forms of governance. The MAP's application of the multisectoral approach has been an effective form of governance in the widespread involvement of people within the HIV/AIDS response, and demonstrated that channelling international aid to the grassroot can be possible. However, the MAP's form of multisectorality reflects the unaccountable unrepresentative side of HIV/AIDS governance. While multiple groups participate within the multisectoral approach to the epidemic, the levels of their involvement are centred on service delivery only; they are not fully represented within decision-making. Furthermore, while groups that receive funds are accountable to the government NACs and DACs, this accountability is not reciprocated by either the government or the Bank. Problems of accountability and representation stem from the structure of the MAP, the contradiction between the NACs 'owning' the MAP and the Bank's use of conditional lending. These problems stem from the wider institutional structures of the Bank and its approach to community-driven, comprehensive development.

The implementation of the World Bank's form of multisectorality through the MAP generates the following conclusions about accountability and participation within HIV/AIDS governance. First, HIV/AIDS governance is still a top-down form of power in which international organisations are able to set the global agenda and instruct governments what to do through conditionalities. This form of governance is justified by reasserting the lack of government leadership within HIV/AIDS that has existed prior to interventions such as the MAP, and the 'expertise' of international organisations such as the Bank. Second, this top-down approach is met with a bottom-up form of accountability. Accountability within the governance of HIV/AIDS goes from communities, national NGOs and governments to international organisations, with little reciprocity. Accountability within HIV/AIDS governance is thus one-sided and biased. Third, the same bias can be applied to participation. Participation within HIV/AIDS governance means implementation and service delivery for community groups and national NGOs; civil society dialogue as a consensual form of decision-making; and the predominance of international actors within agenda-setting and decision-making. As such, the governance of HIV/AIDS is skewed in a way that participation and accountability counts only so far as it implements a form of multisectorality that is preferential to those who define it.

Notes

1 Anonymous quote from a representative of National Council of Women in Kenya

2 Taken from an interview with Nadeem Mohammed, AIDS Campaign Team Africa, World Bank 24th April 2006; this was a response to the question of how the Bank encourages the National AIDS Councils to work with civil society organisations

3 The findings of the chapter are drawn from 163 semi-structured interviews, 50 questionnaires, participant observation of community meetings and partnership forums, findings from an online community forum, and experiences from establishing a UK and Tanzanian based charity, conducted over the course of six months fieldwork between 2005–2006 in Kenya, Tanzania, Uganda, US

4 This was clear in interviews with: Ursula Bahati (National AIDS Control Council Kenya), 14th November 2005; Julius Byenka (Uganda HIV/AIDS Commission), 11th October 2005; Adam Lagerstedt 16th November 2006 (Senior Health Specialist, World Bank Kenya); Emmanuel Malangalila (World Bank Task Team Leader, MAP Tanzania) 20th January 2006.

5 This was clear in conversations with multiple community groups and NGOs, specifically in relation to the MAP. Most groups suggested that funding was coming from USAID and international NGOs.

6 Of the three countries considered – Kenya, Tanzania and Uganda – the strategic plans of each of these three countries echoed the central tenets of the MAP

Bibliography

ACT Africa (2006). Turning Bureaucrats into Warriors: Preparing and Implementing the Multisector HIV-AIDS Programs in Africa: A Generic Operations Manual Washington, DC: World Bank.

Harman, Sophie (2007). 'The World Bank: Failing the Multi-Country AIDS Program, Failing HIV/AIDS' *Global Governance* 13(4): 485–492.

National AIDS Control Council (NACC) (2005a). *Draft Operational Manual: Total War Against HIV/AIDS (TWOA) Project* Nairobi: NACC.

—— (2005b). *Kenya National HIV/AIDS Strategic Plan (KNASP) 2005/6–2009/10: A Call to Action* Nairobi: NACC.

—— (2005c). *Joint AIDS Programme Review 2005 Report* Nairobi: NACC.

Seckinelgin, H. (2005). 'A global disease and its governance: HIV/AIDS in Sub-Saharan Africa and the agency of NGOs' *Global Governance* 11(3): 351–68.

—— (2008). *International Politics of HIV/AIDS: Global Disease – Local Pain* London: Routledge.

Stiglitz, J. (2003). 'Democratizing the IMF and the World Bank: Governance and Accountability,' *Governance* 16(1): 111–39.

TACAIDS (2004). *1st National Multisectoral HIV/AIDS Response Technical Review: Draft Report* Dar es Salaam: TACAIDS.

TACAIDS and GTZ (2005). *Facilitation Notes for the CSO Mapping and Capacity Assessment Tool* Dar es Salaam: TACAIDS.

Tanzania Parliamentarians AIDS Coalition (2004). *Tanzania: Multisectoral AIDS Project (TMAP): Update Sheet 1* Dar es Salaam: Central Printing Works.

Uganda AIDS Commission (2004a). *Draft Report on Mid-Term Review of Uganda HIV/AIDS Control Project* Kampala: UAC.

—— (2004b). *Post-Mid-Term Review Progress Report to World Bank Mission of November 1st to 5th, 2004* Kampala: UAC.

—— (2004c). *UACP HIV/AIDS Annual District Level Workplan* Kampala: UAC.

—— (2005a). *Progress Report to the World Bank Mission of May 2nd to13th, 2005* Kampala: UAC.

—— (2005b). *Progress Report to the Joint Government of Uganda and World Bank Mission of October 3rd to 7th, 2005* Kampala: UAC.

UNAIDS (2005a). *The 'Three Ones' in action: where we are and where we go from here* Geneva: UNAIDS.

—— (2005b). *Global Task Team: on improving AIDS coordination among multilateral institutions and international donors* Geneva: UNAIDS.

United Nations Development Programme (UNDP). (accessed 2008) 'Governance of HIV/AIDS' *http://www.undp.org/hiv/focus02.htm*

UN General Assembly (2001). *UN General Assembly Special Session on HIV/AIDS (UNGASS): Declaration of Commitment on HIV/AIDS* New York: UN.

—— (2006). *2006 High-Level Meeting on AIDS: Uniting the World against AIDS (UNGASS 2006)* New York: UNAIDS.

World Bank (2000a). 'Uganda – HIV/AIDS Control Project: Project Appraisal Document' http://wwwwds.worldbank.org/servlet/WDSContentServer/WDSP/IB/2001/01/26/000094946_01010505342442/Rendered/PDF/multi_page.pdf

—— (2000b). 'Kenya – Decentralised Reproductive Health and HIV/AIDS: Project Appraisal Document' http://wwwwds.worldbank.org/servlet/WDSContentServer/WDSP/IB/2000/12/20/000094946_00112305412221/Rendered/PDF/multi_page.pdf

—— (2000c). 'Kenya – Decentralised Reproductive Health and HIV/AIDS: Project Information Document' http://wwwwds.worldbank.org/servlet/WDSContentServer/WDSP/IB/2000/06/15/000094946_00061505322832/Rendered/PDF/multi0page.pdf

—— (2000d). 'Kenya – HIV/AIDS Disaster Response Project: Project Information Document' http://wwwwds.worldbank.org/servlet/WDSContentServer/WDSP/IB/2000/07/08/000094946_00070706145866/Rendered/PDF/multi0page.pdf

—— (2000e). 'Kenya – HIV/AIDS Disaster Response Project: Project Appraisal Document' http://wwwwds.worldbank.org/servlet/WDSContentServer/WDSP/IB/2000/10/21/000094946_00082605465154/Rendered/PDF/multi_page.pdf272

—— (2000f). *Consultations with Civil Society Organisations: General Guidelines for World Bank Staff* Washington: World Bank
—— (2001). 'Uganda – HIV/AIDS Control Project' http://wwwwds.worldbank.org/servlet/WDSContentServer/WDSP/IB/2000/10/25/000094946_00102505342217/Rendered/PDF/multi0page.pdf
—— (2003a). 'Tanzania – Multi Sectoral AIDS project: Updated Project Information Document' http://wwwwds.worldbank.org/servlet/WDSContentServer/WDSP/IB/2003/07/08/000094946_03062104112344/Rendered/PDF/multi0page.pdf
—— (2003b). 'Tanzania – Multi Sectoral AIDS project: Project Appraisal Document' http://wwwds.worldbank.org/servlet/WDSContentServer/WDSP/IB/2003/06/23/000012009_20030623113128/Rendered/PDF/25761.pdf
—— (2003c). 'Tanzania – Multi Sectoral AIDS project: Environmental Assessment' http://wwwwds.worldbank.org/servlet/WDSContentServer/WDSP/IB/2003/05/23/000094946_03051404055513/Rendered/PDF/multi0page.pdf
—— (2003d). 'Tanzania – Multi Sectoral AIDS project: Integrated Safeguards Data Sheet' http://wwwwds.worldbank.org/servlet/WDSContentServer/WDSP/IB/2001/11/28/000094946_01112104010494/Rendered/PDF/multi0page.pdf
—— (2003e). 'Tanzania – Second Health Sector Development Project: Environmental Assessment' http://wwwwds.worldbank.org/servlet/WDSContentServer/WDSP/IB/2003/10/27/000012009_20031027171627/Rendered/PDF/E812.pdf
—— (2005). *The World Bank's Global HIV/AIDS Program of Action* Washington: World Bank.
—— (2007a). CDF http://web.worldbank.org/WBSITE/EXTERNAL/PROJECTS/STRATEGIES/CDF/0,pagePK:60447~theSitePK:140576,00.html
—— (2007b). PRSP http://web.worldbank.org/WBSITE/EXTERNAL/TOPICS/EXTPOVERTY/EXTPRS/0,menuPK:384207~pagePK:149018~piPK:149093~theSitePK:384201,00.html
—— (2007c). 'The World Bank and Civil Society' http://web.worldbank.org/WBSITE/EXTERNAL/TOPICS/CSO/0,pagePK:220469~theSitePK:228717,00.html
—— (2007d). 'Community Driven Development'http://web.worldbank.org/WBSITE/EXTERNAL/TOPICS/EXTSOCIALDEVELOPMENT/EXTCDD/0,menuPK:430167~pagePK:149018~piPK:149093~theSitePK:430161,00.html
—— (2007e). *The Africa Multi-Country AIDS Program 2000–2006* Washington, DC: World Bank
—— (2008). *The World Bank's Commitment to HIV/AIDS in Africa: Our Agenda for Action, 2007–2011* Washington, DC: World Bank.

Interviews

Gavyole, Awene. 13th February 2006. WHO – Tanzania
Kalinga, Hashim. 14th February 2006. TACAIDS – Tanzania
Kataka, Hanningtone. 23rd November 2005. KUSCCO – Kenya
Kiirya, Stephen. 11th April 2005. Uganda HIV/AIDS Commission – Uganda
Lagerstedt, Adam. 16th November 2005. World Bank – Kenya
Masika, Peter. 13th January 2006. TAYOA – Tanzania
Mohammed, Nadeem. 24th April 2006. World Bank – Washington DC, USA
Namatou, Mary. 20th October 2005. CAWODISA – Uganda
Ngugi, Suzan. 24th November 2005. KENWA – Kenya

Okatcha, Kathleen. 16th November 2005. KORDP – Kenya
Otundo, Kennedy. 28th October 2005. Family Planning Association of Uganda – Uganda
Talugende, Patience. 19th October 2005. ISESWU – Uganda
Wambiya, Paschal. 19th December 2005. ILO – Kenya
Zewdie, Debrework. 3rd May 2006. World Bank – Washington DC, USA

Conclusion

Challenge and Innovation in Governance of HIV/AIDS

Franklyn Lisk

This book has addressed four central questions of governance with regards to HIV/AIDS response:

- What are the major governance requirements and challenges in responding to HIV/AIDS?
- Who are the key actors involved and how effective have their actions been in confronting these challenges?
- What types of structures and mechanisms are required for governance of HIV/AIDS response?
- What changes and innovations are needed for improved governance of HIV/AIDS response?

The discussions and analyses in the preceding chapters have all together offered critical and useful practical insights in providing answers to these questions. They have also identified gaps and deficits in existing governance structures and mechanisms and related institutional arrangements, thereby indicating the need for change and innovation in the governance of HIV/AIDS.

The world of HIV/AIDS, and the response to the epidemic, has changed significantly since the disease was first diagnosed a quarter of a century ago. Over this period, HIV/AIDS has evolved, from a public health condition and a personal tragedy affecting a relatively small number of people within specific groups, into a major global epidemic with potentially devastating economic and social consequences and serious security implications. Both in terms of the numbers infected and those killed by the disease worldwide thus far, HIV/AIDS can be considered as one of the worst humanitarian crises in the history of public health. Similarly, the response to HIV/AIDS has experienced significant developments and major changes during this period: a multiplicity of stakeholders have appeared on the scene and at all levels, from global through regional to national and down to the local community; unique partnerships, institutions, and the extraordinary mobilization of civil society have emerged within countries, across regions and extended right up to the international system; billions of dollars have been raised from various sources for the response, equivalent to the largest amount of money directed at a single health condition so far. The advent of antiretroviral (ARV) drugs for the treatment of AIDS has dramatically transformed HIV/AIDS treatment and care by introducing the possibility of extended lives for people infected with HIV and suffering from AIDS-related illnesses.

All of these developments and changes in the evolution of HIV/AIDS and in its response over the past two decades have impacted on the governance challenge of managing the epidemic at both national and global levels. At the national level, the governance of HIV/AIDS has swiftly escalated from a public health challenge into an unparalleled development challenge, especially in instances where the impact of the epidemic has reversed valuable development gains in health and indicators of development and in effect put a brake on progress towards long-term sustainable development. The evolution of HIV/AIDS into a global HIV/AIDS crisis has been accompanied by a complex global governance challenge, focused on the governance structures and mechanisms of major global institutions whose decisions and actions affect the capacities of developing countries to respond effectively to the epidemic; this challenge has acquired an even larger dimension in an era of globalisation.

Challenges: Multiplicity and complexity of the governance of HIV/AIDS

The issues analysed in the preceding chapters reflect the multiplicity and complexity of the governance of HIV/AIDS which underline the enormous challenge of HIV/AIDS governance at national and international levels. This enormity of the challenge is compounded by the 'exceptionality' of HIV/AIDS, in terms of the mode and speed of transmission of the virus; the deadly impact and wider economic and social consequences; the human rights, legal and ethical implications associated with stigma and discrimination; the amplified gender (inequality) dimensions; the unprecedented international attention backed by the large amount of money from various sources going into fighting this single disease; and yet its continuing evolution and expansion globally, making it a long-wave event with no end in sight. There is now agreement within the international community that the system of governance for managing HIV/AIDS at both global and national levels is crucial to the effectiveness of the response to the epidemic (UNDP 2007; Lisk 2008)

At the same time, interpreting the concept of governance as a 'social contract' between governments and their populations, HIV/AIDS has challenged the responsibility of governments in high prevalence countries for ensuring highest possible standard of public health – as implied in notion of 'the right to health' – and providing protection against the transmission and spread of infectious in their populations. In a wider development context, HIV/AIDS has challenged the responsibility of the state for commitments made within the framework of the Millennium Development Goals (MDGs) to reduce poverty and to achieve long term sustainable development. It has also challenged as the orthodoxy of international development as it relates a reduction of the gap between rich and poor countries over time.

Hence, the link between governance and HIV/AIDS should be analyzed as a 'two-way' bi-directional relationship: the impact of governance on HIV/AIDS response, and the impact of HIV/AIDS on governance capacity. The analyses in the preceding chapters have dealt with both directions of the relationship. They have addressed the type of governance structures and mechanisms required or harmful for effective HIV/AIDS response (chapters by Handley, Hayes, Lisk, Sutherland and Potts), and have also drawn attention to how the erosion of governance capacity linked to impact of HIV/AIDS could undermine economic growth, social progress and political stability (chapters by Kondwani and Hatendi-Gutu).

Throughout the developing regions, and particularly in Sub-Saharan Africa where the impact of the epidemic has been most severe, governments are faced with an increasingly difficult task of responding to the exceptional proportions and the complexities of the HIV/AIDS crisis. The epidemic has impoverished families and communities, and has resulted in social exclusion and countless human rights violations. It has also heightened existing gender inequalities, as women and girls are particularly vulnerable to HIV and disproportionately affected. Such is the threat that the epidemic poses to sustainable development, that HIV/AIDS has been identified by the United Nations and the international community as a major obstacle to the achievement of the Millennium Development Goals (MDGs) for many developing countries.

The main challenge faced in HIV/AIDS governance at the global level concerns the effects of imbalances and distortions in the current system of global governance. This can be a drawback on the capacity of highly affected and other developing countries to respond effectively to the epidemic and its impact on their economies and populations. The focus is on the governance structures of global institutions that make or influence decisions pertaining to intellectual property rights and access to ARV drugs; regulation of global financial flows and external debt transactions; and macro-economic frameworks for sustained HIV/AIDS financing. The fact that decision-making authority in institutions such as the World Trade Organisations (WTO), World Bank and the International Monetary Fund (IMF) is dominated and controlled by the rich countries of the global North relative to the influence of the poorer ones of the South is a major governance challenge, especially as decisions made are perceived to restrict access of developing countries to essential life-extending HIV/AIDS medicines and additional financial resources needed to boost their HIV/AIDS response efforts.

Response: Change and innovation in the governance of HIV/AIDS

The great and growing challenge of HIV/AIDS governance suggests that more attention should be given to this issue in the wider context of the response to the epidemic at all levels. There is consensus within the UN and international community that effective governance is essential for an effective response to HIV/AIDS (UNDP 2007). Key elements of governance, such as participation, representation, legitimacy, accountability and transparency are deemed critical to global and national efforts to address HIV/AIDS, all the more so when we take into account the large number of different stakeholders and interests involved and the substantial cash flows that go into the response.

At the national level, the notion of governance in relation to HIV/AIDS response implies first and foremost the broadening of *participation* in the formulation and implementation of strategies, policies and programmes to combat the epidemic. The requirement goes beyond the model of a government-led process, which could be end up being a 'top-down' arrangement which can be fraught with the danger of social inequalities and inefficiencies as highlighted in Sutherland's chapter on recent Chinese experience in HIV/AIDS governance. What is also needed is a 'bottom-up' approach centred on the active involvement of civil society organisations, especially at the community level, in the planning and delivery of HIV/AIDS services and for monitoring of local authorities policy and action in the response, as illustrated in the Kenyan case study presented in Shannon Hayes' chapter. Local-level, broad-based participation, including importantly those affected through infection and caring for family members, is required for identifying and prioritising needs of the community and ensuring that the response is accordingly directed at those needs, and that the process is as transparent as possible.

It is now evident that the social partners of government at the country level can also contribute significantly to improved governance of HIV/AIDS response. In the context of many highly affected countries the domestic private sector and business in particular had been at the forefront of the response even before the government was empowered through external financial support to take action. Antoinette Handley's chapter on the role of business in the response in South Africa depicts the importance of this contribution for governance, but at the same time makes it clear that action by firms also stemmed from concern about the impact of the epidemic on their businesses. The role of the private sector as a partner of the state, rather than an independent stakeholder, in fighting HIV/AIDS has brought into prominence the notion of public-private partnership (PPP) as a practical mechanism for improving governance and thereby contributing to a more effective response to the epidemic. In such a partnership, it is important that there is a balance between the interest of the state and the needs of the private sector, including the distinction of needs between employers and labour, as illustrated and analysed in the chapter by Franklyn Lisk.

Good governance also implies the need for *accountability* with respect to oversight on how resources are allocated and spent, and the impact of HIV/AIDS expenditure (Lisk 2006b). It is important to bear in mind that accountability has to be reciprocal, in terms of the need for recipient governments and external donors to hold each other accountable for the implementation and impact of programmes – a requirement which comes out clearly in Hatendi-Gutu's chapter on the operations of the Global Fund to Fight AIDS, Tuberculosis and Malaria (Global Fund) in Zimbabwe. Government's accountability to stakeholders can be advanced through various means, such as creating action-oriented and time-bound agenda linked to clearly defined and measurable targets; publishing and disseminating audited reports; and setting up an independent and representative monitoring and evaluation mechanism to review and assess HIV/AIDS programmes and interventions periodically. Also fundamental to the notion of accountability in the context of HIV/AIDS response is the responsibility of the state to ensure the right to the highest attainable standard health for all citizens as a pre-requisite for good governance, that is the focus of Helen Potts' chapter. In this regard, there is an important role for government and parliament in making laws and putting in place the legal and policy framework for managing HIV/AIDS and promoting the right to health. Kondwani Chirambo's chapter, however, shows that deadly impact of the epidemic on the law makers themselves and on the electoral process is a major challenge that must be addressed in a comprehensive response. One might go as far as to suggest that, from the standpoint of governance, members of the government and parliamentarians as leaders and elected representatives of the people have a special responsibility to set examples that will inspire others to take appropriate action to protect themselves and their families from the risk of HIV infection. This type of leadership quality denotes moral authority that can be considered an integral component of accountability.

At the global level, the democratic deficit in global governance between the North and South is derived mainly from structures and arrangements that may no longer be relevant to the realities of present-day global geo-political and economic relations. Hence, there are demands from the developing countries and their supporters in the international community for a re-examination of the current system of global governance, and the need to redress the balance of power between the North and South by giving more voice and influence to South. In the specific context of HIV/AIDS, a new architecture of global governance as called for by developing countries would not only improve their capacity to respond more effectively to HIV/AIDS challenges, but will be commensurate with the substantive importance of the global HIV/AIDS crisis in the international agenda, particularly the MDGs (Lisk 2008).

The inadequacy of existing institutional arrangements governing international flows of trade, finance and investments calls for change and innovation in both the ideas and institutions of the system of global governance. However, change and innovation in the system of global governance must be linked to improvement in democratic governance at the national level, since the latter also affects the capacity of countries to respond effectively to the HIV/AIDS epidemic. For example, change in global governance resulting in debt relief and the mobilization of additional financial resources for HIV/

AIDS response must go hand in hand with the efficient and transparent use of funds at the country level. Similarly, reduction in the costs of ARV drugs as a result of greater flexibility in the application of intellectual property rights and trade agreements at global level need to be complemented by the responsibility of governments at country level to provide of adequate health infrastructure and delivery systems for ensuring access. This leads to the conclusion that the capacities of developing countries to respond effectively to HIV/AIDS also require adequate space for sound democratic governance.

Sophie Harman's analysis of governance of HIV/AIDS from the perspective of interventions by the World Bank – an institution that is often the target of criticisms from the developing countries and international NGOs about the negative impact of its policies and programmes on development capacity – shows that the Bank has actually made a significant contribution to improvement in HIV/AIDS governance at national level through its Multi-Country AIDS Program (MAP), which involves the participation of civil society organisations in partnership with governments in many highly affected countries. Harman's chapter provides evidence of the need to take account of linkages between global governance and national-level governance in any new architecture of global governance for HIV/AIDS response. Finally, an important requirement of global governance as regards the overall relationship between global financial and economic institutions and developing countries, is recognition by those institutions of the need for a balance between economic and social objectives in their policy prescriptions and country programmes. This will go a long way towards helping poorer countries to respond better and more effectively to development challenges like HIV/AIDS.

Bibliography

Harman, S. (2007). "Operational and policy implementation framework for HIV/AIDS response" *UNDP/CSGR University of Warwick, Working Paper 3.* UNDP, New York March 2007.

ILO (2003). "Global compact policy dialogue on HIV/AIDS: Meeting Report", ILO/AIDS, Geneva May 2003.

Lisk, F. (2006a). "Global governance and HIV/AIDS response", *UNDP/CSGR University of Warwick, Working Paper 1.* UNDP, New York December 2006.

—— (2006b). "National governance and HIV/AIDS response", *UNDP/CSGR University of Warwick, Working Paper 2.* UNDP, New York December 2006.

—— (2008). "Towards a new architecture of global governance for responding to the HIV/AIDS epidemic" in A. Cooper, B. Hocking and W. Maley (eds) *Global governance and Diplomacy: Worlds apart.* Basingstoke: Palgrave Macmillan.

UNDP (2006). *Corporate strategy on HIV/AIDS.* UNDP, New York.

—— (2007). Governance and HIV/AIDS responses: Issues and outlook. UNDP, New York.

Index

For Product Safety Concerns and Information please contact our EU representative GPSR@taylorandfrancis.com
Taylor & Francis Verlag GmbH, Kaufingerstraße 24, 80331 München, Germany

www.ingramcontent.com/pod-product-compliance
Lightning Source LLC
LaVergne TN
LVHW011131300926
849160LV00008B/601

9780415848022